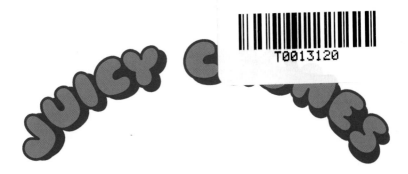

FREE FOR THE
STRANGEST ADVENTURES

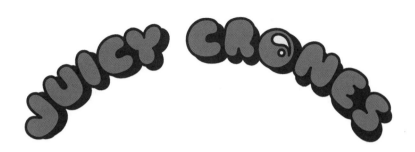

JUICY CRONES

FREE FOR THE STRANGEST ADVENTURES

INSPIRATIONAL STORIES OF WOMEN EMBRACING LATER LIFE

JAY COURTNEY

Bradt GUIDES

First published in the UK in January 2023 by
Bradt Guides Ltd
31a High Street, Chesham, HP5 1BW, England
www.bradtguides.com

Print edition published in the USA by The Globe Pequot Press Inc,
PO Box 480, Guilford, Connecticut 06437-0480

Edited by Samantha Cook
Cover design by Laura Greenan/IllustrationX
Layout and typesetting by Ian Spick, Bradt Guides
Production managed by Sue Cooper, Bradt Guides & Zenith Media

ISBN: 9781784779573

British Library Cataloguing in Publication Data
A catalogue record for this book is available from the British Library

Digital conversion by www.dataworks.co.in
Printed in the UK by Zenith Media

To my powerful and beautiful daughters,
and my wonderful and magical granddaughters.
My wish for you is that, by the time you become crones, you
will wonder what I was making such a fuss about.
With immense love and gratitude to you all.

CONTENTS

PREFACE

For now she need not think about anybody. She could be herself, by herself. And that was what now she often felt the need of – to think; well, not even to think. To be silent; to be alone. All the being and the doing, expansive, glittering, vocal, evaporated; and one shrunk, with a sense of solemnity, to being oneself, a wedge-shaped core of darkness, something invisible to others. Although she continued to knit, and sat upright, it was thus that she felt herself; and this self having shed its attachments was free for the strangest adventures.

Virginia Woolf, *To the Lighthouse*

The germ of this book started to grow when I retired. I was finding my way into a different life from the world of work and family that I had known for almost forty years. Those years were gone, and I was afraid that I had too. It was an exciting time, daunting, and sometimes challenging, to keep what the poet Dorothy Nimmo described as the 'black parrots' at bay: those squawking voices that tell us we are too old, too wrinkly, and so on. It was, and still is, a time to wrestle with the big questions of life, death and meaning, but most of all to give myself permission to live this part of my life to the full. Virginia Woolf's phrase 'free for the strangest adventures' lodged itself as an earworm – in the words of my friend Gilly, there are only two stages in life: '*not* too late and *too* late'. I needed to get a wriggle on.

I did not have a true notion of what it meant to be an older woman, not least because I couldn't identify with any of the labels: post-menopausal (ugh), retiree (even the word sounds like 'tired'), pensioner (double ugh), a woman in her third act (hmm?), old witch (getting warmer!), second spring-er (do I like it?), glamorous granny (oh God, back to being defined by how we look and who we are related to)... And then there's 'crone'. I always used to recoil from that as a way to describe an older woman. But psychologist Jean Shinoda Bolen, laughing in the face of this descriptor with her 'Juicy Crone' epithet, encouraged me to embrace it – and the term still makes me smile. It is likely that the word crone is a corruption of 'crown', referring to our crowning years of wisdom and knowledge. Honour and respect the crown!

At the start, mine was not a conscious quest – I was simply hoping to travel and have fun, try new things outside my comfort zone and study new subjects. It had overtones of those first heady days of leaving home for student life and feeling anything was possible, albeit with a wiser head, a broader beam and more money in my pocket. And, as I ventured forth, I was enjoying meeting other women who were similarly seeking enlightenment about what life post-menopause might mean for them. I began to realise that adventures come in many guises, often in the most unexpected form, and often starting from a place of inner conflict.

The more women I spoke to, the more I realised that I wasn't alone in my struggle – other women were wrestling with questions of meaning and purpose, too.

I learned that many were living remarkable lives, and I decided to ask them if they would be willing to share their stories. I was seeking women who, like myself, had jobs or responsibilities that came to a defined or perhaps abrupt end due to ill health, redundancy or bereavement, or because of new caring responsibilities. Or women who had nursed a long-held ambition and came the day when they decided, if not now, then when? Luckily, many women were glad to speak to me. As I listened, talked and recorded their accounts, I was, without realising it, writing the book that I had wanted to read.

After all the other 'isms' I had faced in my life, ageism was the most unexpected and, in many ways, damaging. In the period that the *Juicy Crones* project started to take shape, I was growing new wings and starting to fly in different directions. While it could feel a bit crazy, sometimes demeaning, it was also exciting and entertaining to challenge and dispel myths. And then, just as I was trying to discard (or at least let slip a little) the metaphorical masks that were no longer serving me, all of a sudden we were required by law to wear physical masks because of the Covid-19 pandemic. Evidence began to emerge that wearing a mask might not do much to protect the wearer but offered protection to other people, especially when coupled with the two-metre distance rule. Had I all these years worn metaphoric masks to protect myself or others, I wondered?

Ironically *Juicy Crones: Free for the Strangest Adventures* was written mostly during this period of severe restriction. International travel was curtailed and for several months I was, like everyone else, tethered to my home. My first outing was to the dentist. Who would have imagined that would ever feel like 'going out'? Sometimes I could laugh at the irony of writing my first book with the subtitle 'Free for the Strangest Adventures' at this time – and sometimes it led me into the depths of despair. Writing the book during the pandemic meant it became a different type of project, a strange adventure in itself, meeting women – in real life and virtually – I would not otherwise have met. The gravity and intensity of the pandemic sharpened our focus onto what mattered most, and this is now reflected in our ambition for cronehood.

This is not a self-help book, but I hope the riches of the twelve women who share their stories here do help you, that they reassure you that you are not alone in your journey, and that they challenge you to find your own unique way of becoming a Juicy Crone. I also hope that, in that wonderful way of women, you in turn can inspire, support and aid other women as they too find their way. I'm calling these women 'cronees' – our sisters-in-arms, there to give each other an unfair advantage in our quest to be juicy.

I wish you well in your journey whether you are female or no, in your third act or not yet. For me: Oh, I am just getting started!

1

ATROPHY, ENTROPY

The word 'anti-ageing' has to be struck. I am pro-ageing. I want to age with intelligence, and grace, and dignity, and verve and energy.
Jamie Lee Curtis, Radically Reframing Aging Summit, 2022

'It's vaginal atrophy.'

'What do you mean? My insides are dying?'

'Not dying. Just not quite what they were. It's very common at your age.'

'At your age' becomes the prefix or suffix to each and every consultation with a medical professional after this day. Mostly I learn to ignore this received wisdom and defy the ageist remarks. But this first time, I am taken aback.

'Is there a cure?' I ask.

'Not a cure, but I can prescribe something that should help. My ladies tell me that it keeps their husbands happy.'

Good to know.

How had I never heard of this happening to women? The pain on sitting, walking, in fact just *being*, let alone anything friskier. We all know about men and their little blue pills. Even mainstream television carries adverts for erectile dysfunction, where toned, handsome, athletic older men pop a little blue pill – and everyone is smiling again. I was quite sure I had never seen anything in the adverts about vaginal atrophy. Why is the descriptor 'atrophy' used of women but 'dysfunction' of men? Are women of a certain age simply on a point of collapse, disintegrating by the day, whereas men just need a little pharmacological engineering to get them fully functioning again? Do men have the potential to be indefinitely virile while women are in a state of steady decay? I had never seen anyone with a wink-wink and a nudge-nudge discussing the older woman's hapless situation with painful sex. I don't get the impression that the pharmaceutical industry is busting a gut to ensure that women can pop a pink pill to feel aroused and potent again. Adverts are not written for women to celebrate pleasure for pleasure's sake now that we are past the point of being useful and producing babies.

At home, I rush to consult Dr Google. Had I misheard? Had she (the real doctor) said atrophy or entropy?

Atrophy. Verb: 'Physical or psychological decline.' Noun: 'Weakening due to lack of use.'

Entropy. Noun: 'Uncertainty or disorder in the system. The gradual breakdown of energy and matter in the universe. Degradation, disorder.'

The medical definition of 'atrophy' is 'decrease in size or wasting away of a body part or tissue'. But I didn't know that then. I pause for a while, sitting on my atrophied insides. Perhaps it was while my insides atrophied that my world entropied? Or perhaps the causation went the other way? Like most women, my pre-atrophied insides have experienced menstruation, sex, procreation, birthing and, latterly, menopause. Are we, in the words of Margaret Atwood in *The Handmaid's Tale*, simply 'two-legged wombs'? Was menopause the end of *me*? Was my body mourning the end of its reproductive faculty? My mind certainly wasn't. I love my children and grandchildren dearly – they bring joy to me every day. Choosing to bring new life into the world and nurturing it well is demanding and incredibly rewarding, but I had no regrets about the end of my childbearing years and was glad and relieved to say goodbye to the messy, painful, uncomfortable business of menstruation. I was relieved to no longer be sabotaged every month by a tsunami of hormones that swept me high and plummeted me to the depths. Was this where the fault line in my understanding lay? Was I so buffeted by menopausal symptoms that I was struggling to right myself? Was my body weak due to lack of use or simply exhausted and needing a good holiday, like the rest of me? Was it taking its own last stand against the disorder in the universe? Or was it, perhaps, that I had no post-menopausal role models to aspire to and couldn't see beyond my decline? From where I was sitting, all these thoughts resonated.

This visit to my doctor happened when I was in my early fifties, ten or so years ago. So little was talked about menopause publicly then, especially in the work environment, that I knew very little of what to expect. We had to muddle through as best we could. I was reminded of my periods starting all those years before and my mother's main concern being that I shouldn't leave anything lying around to offend my father or brothers. It seemed that this was another major life transition for a woman that should be neither seen nor heard, something shaming. A dirty secret. There seemed to be a collusion of silence.

Things are changing now, thank goodness. Television programmes have been aired about the menopause, many books have been written and there are social media sites to support perimenopausal and menopausal health. There is an increasing recognition that there isn't a one-size-fits-all solution to women's health, and we are learning more about how our gut health can help us stay well, especially to support our immune system and rebalance hormones. However, in women-centred health provision, there is a long way to go.

Arguably the most offensive word in the English language refers to the most central, pleasure-giving, life-affirming, life-giving, extraordinary part of the female anatomy – not just an offensive, rude word, but an obscene word. Women's bodies have been denigrated and commodified throughout history. No wonder, then, that we often have deeply conflicted feelings about our bodies and deny ourselves the deep pleasures and life force to be found there. The only commodification my body seemed to be attracting was promises of eye-wateringly expensive age-defying creams and potions. Heaven forbid that I should look like I have been alive for over fifty years: denigration now came in more subtle forms, and from the attitudes of the medical profession.

Things have come to a pretty pass.

Atrophy, entropy.

Let's call the whole thing off.

Something must be done.

But what?

Until that day I had always been working *towards* something: completing my education, raising my children, building my career, fixing broken houses, fighting homophobia – just living my life in the face of opposition and inequality. I hadn't noticed that the outward and visible signs were announcing my demise. But apparently the inward, invisible signs were telling their story. I was in decline, decay. Longevity runs in my family – with any luck I would make it into my late eighties or early nineties. The thought of thirty years of entropy (or was it atrophy – I still couldn't work it out) was disturbing and disappointing. Having worked so hard all my life to be an independent woman – a full person – I was in real danger of that being written off. I was older, no longer fertile and therefore expendable.

I needed to get a grip. I needed to get a life – a post-menopausal life.

No more decay – eyes towards rejuvenation. Was there a pessary for that?

Just after my atrophy diagnosis, I returned from a holiday in Greece with a nasty infection, possibly swine flu. Wiped out by it, I just couldn't seem to shake it off. I probably went back to work too soon and then got one infection after another. After many false starts, I couldn't sustain a return to work. It felt as if neither my body nor my mind was under my control. My limbs felt like they were drugged – I could no longer run, or even walk fast. I wasn't confident that I would be able to jump out of the way of an oncoming lorry. I had always swum at the gym every morning before work, but now just getting into my swimsuit was exhausting and it took all my energy to haul myself out of the pool, let alone swim.

For several weeks the doctor entered 'Malaise' on my sick note. After months of living in this limbo I pressed her for a diagnosis. She said, 'I can put down CFS if you really want to go down that route.' I had no idea what that meant.

Diagnosing chronic fatigue syndrome (CFS), or myalgic encephalitis (ME), is an imprecise science. There is no blood test for it; instead, once you have had a cluster of certain common symptoms for six months or so, with no real sign of things getting better, you will likely end up being diagnosed with CFS or ME or post-viral fatigue. It was not reassuring that the diagnosis was vague and that the medical profession could not even agree on what to name it.

I had no energy, no drive. I was indecisive and struggled to complete simple daily tasks. I was constantly getting colds and coughs. My lungs frequently felt congested and infected, but visits to the GP usually resulted in the doctor telling me that my lungs sounded clear. I was often breathless and wheezed my way into strategic meetings. My GP had nothing to offer me except antidepressants. I wasn't depressed, but I was angry and frustrated that almost no research had been done to understand this common condition, let alone treat it.

Chronic fatigue syndrome is one of those illnesses that everyone has an opinion about, but no-one has an answer to, scientific or otherwise. Medical experts are divided between those who think it is psychosomatic and those who believe it is a debilitating post-viral condition and that little is known about how to treat it. Some attribute it to adrenal failure. Others call it 'yuppie flu' – or even (from one of my colleagues, within earshot) 'lazy fucker's disease'. Everyone I consulted gave conflicting advice: I tried everything and none of it really helped. Some things, like graded exercise therapy, made it so much worse and left me feeling like a failure to boot.

I was a woman who set targets and achieved them. But that approach did not work for this illness: it was counterintuitive. I could not help myself and I lost my sense of *me*. Every day for years I woke up feeling that I was coming down with the flu. Every day I tried to rise above it, some days more successfully than others. A big part of my job was making presentations and public speaking – something I was used to. I could still perform well, but the cost to my energy supplies was high and the fallout when I got home devastating.

I was aware that some people with ME/CFS literally faded away and died from it, or lived an existence that, like mine, felt like barely living. Others were sectioned under the Mental Health Act by medics assuming they were suffering from some form of mental illness. Of course it was affecting my mental health – it was literally driving me bloody mad. I felt like a Victorian woman diagnosed with the vapours.

Family occasions, which I had always loved, left me so wiped out in the days afterwards that I had to ration my energy. It hurt me so much not to see as much of my new-born granddaughter as I wanted. Even holding her was at times exhausting.

Frustration uses up a great deal of energy, and learning to accept my state of health without fighting it and being angry was a real life lesson. I was a fighter, a leader – I was terrible at sitting and being patient without something to do. I could hear my mother's voice, 'The devil finds work for idle hands!', imploring me not to be lazy. *Being* wasn't my thing. *Doing* was. I read Tim Parks' book *Teach Us to Sit Still*, about learning Vipassana meditation, and I identified so strongly with his mystery illness that I laughed and cried at his attempts to meditate. Put me in a meditation room at that time, and rather than feeling calmed I would have gone into full-frontal panic.

The specialist advised me to manage my days in chunks of time. She gave me 'energy charts' to monitor my daily activity and rest and how my body responded to both. I was to colour in boxes in five- and fifteen-minute slots. The aim was always to do less than I thought I could. What? I'd fought my whole life not to colour inside the lines and here I was, being advised to do quite literally that – and I hated it. Looking at the charts with their primary-school large print and crayon colouring made me feel that my life had not only lost meaning but it had taken a nose-dive over a cliff.

Finally, several weeks after my diagnosis, my GP managed to get me a place on a specialist course for people suffering from CFS. I was desperate to get advice and solutions. The only problem was that the course – held in the Independent Living Centre, a name I loathed with its unpleasant implication that I was no longer independent, and needed help or aides – was in a small village a two-hour drive from my house, with no public transport. I hit heavy morning traffic en route and arrived after the ten o'clock start.

Late and flustered, I walked into a room where five other ME/CFS sufferers were sitting in a circle listening to a presentation by a health professional. As I settled in, I glanced around the edge of the room: bed pans, bed hoists, walking frames, motorised buggies, adapted furniture, easy-grip cutlery and incontinence aids were all on display. Apart from the deaths of loved ones, it was the lowest point of my life. I had no idea what the presenter was saying – all I could see was an implied vision of the future ahead of me. The only good thing about the whole day was meeting fellow sufferers: three men and two women, all high achievers, many self-made entrepreneurs, all as frustrated and fed up as me, though – unlike me – some of their marriages were not surviving this illness, and one had gone bankrupt because of it. We were sent away with yet more charts to colour in. As I set off to drive home, I realised I could not. One of the symptoms I suffered from was blurred vision when I got tired. I simply did not have the ability or energy to make the journey. I wondered if I would get home at all that day. I took refuge in a garden centre tea shop, napped in the car, and then limped home exhausted and overwhelmed by my prospects. It took several days of bed rest before I could move again.

Looking back now it seems obvious that life had just thrown too much at me all at once: the death of both my parents, the death of close friends, trauma with children. This was 2009, and the financial crisis, as it was euphemistically called, of the previous year had had catastrophic effects on children's services in the local authority where I worked. I was forced by the austerity government to make redundant a whole team of people whose life's work had been dedicated to children's health and well-being, while the bankers still got their bonuses. I was outraged by this but was not allowed to voice it because I worked within a political environment.

The Great Recession (as it became known) was in large part due to excessive financial risk, even fraud, that reverberated throughout the global economy. By the time its effects had reached my small team it had manifested itself in both tragic and occasionally comic results. Three colleagues from the children's health and well-being team, all under the age of sixty, died within the next three years. They had dedicated their careers to improving outcomes for children. It was hard not to see a correlation. They were good friends – the pain was personal as well as professional. I missed them terribly.

Despite draconian budget cuts, we still had targets to reach on the strategic plans. One of these targets was the reduction of unwanted teenage pregnancies. Meanwhile, centres offering young people help with all aspects of health and well-being were forced to reduce their hours while at the same time the budget for physical- and mental-health education in schools was severely cut. There was no longer any money even to buy condoms for demonstration purposes in sex-education lessons. Young people were consequently at risk of unwanted pregnancies and increased rates of sexually transmitted infections. I was so angry about this that I phoned around all the condom manufacturers until one offered to give me some of their stock that was past its Kitemark date. I drove to the manufacturer and loaded the huge boxes, containing 13,500 condoms, into my car. It was a Renault Scenic, which, as its name suggests, has big windows – ideal for displaying to the world what I was carrying. As

I drove, I tried to invent a plausible explanation in case the police stopped me. Nothing really sounded convincing!

I cannot say government policy at the time caused my illness, but it certainly contributed. Stress at work and at home were intolerably high, but I couldn't see it. I became ill with a virus; I didn't listen to my body telling me to rest and I exhausted its natural healing reserves. My body had no resources left for fight or flight and I had left it with only one option: freeze. Self-care 101 – look after your health before it is too late. Put on your own oxygen mask before helping others.

Chronic fatigue resulted in me being off work for almost six months. I took all the help I could get, and through trial and error learned what helped and what didn't. Slowly and painfully, one step at a time, I got closer to returning to work. Occupational Health at my local authority was very supportive and took its directive on ME/CFS from the World Health Organization's guidance. This favoured me with a much longer than usual phased return to work, which in turn enabled me to manage my energy levels very carefully. At the same time my GP told me that my local hospital was now running a course on recovery from ME/CFS, and she made the referral.

I went to the local hospital to meet the nurse who would be running the course. By her own admission she was new to this, didn't know anything about ME/CFS, but was really looking forward to leading the group – and could I just complete the paperwork. By now I was familiar with the drill: any kind of support offered came with the proviso that you filled in reams of questionnaires and lots more colouring-in of boxes. I ploughed through the bureaucracy to get a place. When I reached the last two sets of paperwork, I came across a code that read something like CFS 2306 SAH. Two questions in, I realised what this was code for:

1. Do you consider yourself to be a hypochondriac?
2. Have any members of your family ever described you as
   a hypochondriac?

And so it continued, question after question, attempting to diagnose if I had thought myself into being ill.

I could not believe what I was being asked: I was being asked to self-assess for hypochondria! Hence the 'SAH'. When I questioned the nurse, she shrugged. Had I heard of health anxiety syndrome? I had not. Had she heard of a cancer patient being asked to answer such a question? A schizophrenic? An MS patient? A depressive?

I left.

I don't dispute that the mind can have a powerful effect on our physical well-being – why else would the placebo be the baseline for all drug testing? I knew I needed a positive mindset if I was to recover, but I had come to accept that I needed more than just that. Afterwards, in my research, I learned that before they had a clinical aetiology, many diseases were deemed to be due to hypochondria. The incidence of this was higher where the disease presented more often in women than men. In short, women were 'acting up'. Multiple sclerosis – or hysterical paralysis, as it was called in its early days – was one such disease. Only later did autopsies show the demyelination of the brain and spinal cord that it causes.

According to a 2021 article in the Royal College of Physicians' *Clinical Medicine* journal (w rcpjournals.org/content/clinmedicine/21/1/13), medically unexplained symptoms or persistent physical symptoms account for around twenty per cent of primary care consultations. But not being explainable is not the same as not existing.

Finally, I went to see an endocrinologist. After a thorough examination and extensive blood tests he said, 'I can see you are unwell, you are not imagining it, but the truth is that no-one really knows what causes this. There is just so much we do not know.' His advice was to rest, do nothing that I did not feel like doing, and let my body heal itself. He said some patients had found improvement by cutting simple carbohydrates out of their diet. Rather than feel like the consultation was a waste of money, it was like a breath of fresh air. This was mostly because I felt heard – he believed me and wasn't pretending to know something that just does not have solid research behind it – and partly because he was talking about self-healing. I had always believed in the body's ability to heal itself and I had avoided taking drugs if I possibly could. I felt both relief and hope that, in time, I could recover.

One of the things I tried at this time was the 'Lightning Process', a form of neurolinguistic programming. It was expensive and plenty of people were sceptical about it. I too weighed up if this was snake oil, preying on the vulnerable, but trusted the no-nonsense friends who recommended it. I decided it was worth investing in – and it was. It taught me to control negative thoughts and believe in my own agency. Perversely, living with chronic fatigue takes stamina – to keep positive and hopeful needs mental discipline. It wasn't a miracle cure, but it was one big step towards healing.

I would not wish this illness on anyone, and with so many people globally now suffering from long Covid, we can only hope that post-viral illness will no longer be ignored, and that serious research into its cause and cure will be undertaken. One small trial may be shedding light on post-viral difficulties with breathing; a small study using hyperpolarised Xenon MRI scans has identified previously undetectable abnormalities in the lungs of long Covid patients. I have no means of knowing if the same might be true in my case, but I am relieved to think that my lungs were not in my head. I remember the feeling of not being able to breathe in, as if my lungs had been cauterised. Spike Milligan famously requested the words 'I told you I was ill' on his tombstone. I would like to have the words 'I told you I couldn't breathe' on mine.

Throughout my illness, well-meaning people would say, 'Look after yourself.' I was puzzled. Having spent my professional life on matters relating to health and well-being, why didn't I know what they meant? Then the penny dropped. It wasn't the 'look after' bit I was stuck on – it was the 'self'. Did I know myself at this time in my life? Had I ever really known 'me'? Discovering a renewed sense of self seemed to be at the heart of my recovery from this insidious illness. I had to accept that I couldn't continue with my job for much longer, but I was determined not to finish 'on grounds of ill health', even though financially it would have been the wise thing to do. So, in 2014 I made the difficult decision to retire at the end of the year.

My whole professional career was focused on the well-being of young people. I taught teenagers, and while the gap between our ages widened from just over three years when I was a newly qualified teacher to almost three decades when I became a local authority advisor, I still spent my days listening to the needs and life stories of young people. When the austerity crisis hit in 2008, I had to find a way to resuscitate the Children's Health and Well-Being service, which offered support and advice to all schools in the county. Several headteachers graciously allowed me a temporary transfer of their best teachers for one day a week so that I could create a taskforce to continue to support the welfare of young people. This team was brilliant – during the recession children, families and school budgets suffered badly, but the team were there to help in any way that they could.

By 2014, through a partnership with Foster and Brown Research, we had been listening via confidential, online surveys for ten years to the voices of children and young people from more than three hundred schools, giving us one of the richest data sets of young voices in the world. We asked questions about issues as diverse as leisure activities, bullying and online grooming. One of the specialisms of the team was delivering training to teachers and other professionals and writing resources for use in the classroom. We set ourselves the ambitious goal of writing a ground-breaking curriculum that put the voice of the child at the centre of teaching and learning. Each school's data from the survey enabled their children's voices to directly inform the curriculum, thus matching student needs with the lessons taught. It was a huge undertaking, which the team continued to work on despite my periods of absence. The launch was a very proud moment for us all, and the keynote speech I made at the event was a fitting finale for my career. I could leave with my head held high, feeling I had left a legacy that I could only hope would make a difference to young lives.

Retirement came as much of a shock to me as ill health. I felt dislocated. The transient nature of life was disabling. How was I to put down roots in something which, apart from my pension pot, I had not invested? I had never given retirement a moment's thought – why would I? I loved my work. In fact, it came as a complete shock to me that I was old enough to retire at all. I had colleagues who had a countdown to retirement pinned to their desk. I didn't. Elderly parents retire, friends retire, *other people* retire. Some people dream of giving up work, going on a world cruise, putting their feet up. I didn't. My wife and I travelled extensively and loved it, but I didn't need to retire to do that. Retirement simply wasn't on my agenda. It wasn't about being in denial – it just hadn't occurred to me. Or perhaps I was denying the denial?

The farewell party was over and my colleagues were back at work. I woke up as usual at 6am and thought: now what? It was January 2015, cold and dreary. It wasn't a holiday, and I wasn't ill, although not one hundred per cent well either. I was home alone, and I had absolutely no idea what came next or what I should be doing.

I realised I just did not know how to do this part of my life. Like many career women of my age, I felt invincibility had suddenly been replaced by invisibility. As William James wrote in 1890, in *The Principles of Psychology*:

No more fiendish punishment could be devised, were such a thing physically possible, than that one should be turned loose in society and remain absolutely unnoticed by all the members thereof.

My family still noticed me, but I had lost a huge part of my tribe – my work tribe. And having lost that, the world around me turned greige. I could no longer apply my work mask. I no longer had the scaffolding of titles and positions to hold me up. I had a pervasive feeling of not being real. On paper I was a very lucky woman, but my tree of life was withering and I didn't know why. I could sense I needed a root-and-branch solution, but this would require a different kind of work.

I was not conscious of it at the time, but it was in this rather glum and unprepossessing context that I started my quest.

2

WELL-GROOMED WOMEN

'The reasonable man adapts himself to the world: the unreasonable one persists in trying to adapt the world to himself. Therefore, all progress depends on the unreasonable man.

George Bernard Shaw, 1903'

Or woman.   Helen Lewis, 2020

Helen Lewis, *Difficult Women*

As a very proud grandmother, I watched my granddaughters banging out Robbie Williams' song 'I Love My Life' in their primary school concert. As they strutted their stuff on stage they were urgent, insistent that they were indeed powerful, beautiful, wonderful, magical and FREE. They yelled and they stabbed their fingers: 'I am not my mistakes.' My greatest wish for them is that they internalise this – that when life throws up challenges, this will be their mantra.

It was a bittersweet moment for me: if my childhood friends and I had ever tried to express any of those sentiments we would have been slapped down immediately by home, by school, by church. And as for our mistakes? We were taught that those would be a stain on our character forever.

The Juicy Crones celebrated in this book were born between 1940 and 1965, arguably one of the biggest periods of social and political upheaval in modern history. It's useful to remember that we were born to mothers who were formed between the 1920s and

1940s. It wasn't until I started to write this chapter – to contextualise the era in which the women in this book grew up – that I realised why, when I talk about my childhood and upbringing, my daughters roll their eyes and mutter, 'Mum's off talking about days of yore again.' My daughters have been raised, I hope, to see themselves as equal, independent women with agency, and somewhere along the line I hadn't taken in how much – albeit slowly – women's lives have changed.

As I write this chapter, the anniversary of my mother's birth is approaching; it is always a time of reflection and gratitude for all that she gave to me. Win Courtney was born in 1923 in Walthamstow, the middle child of a large family. Her father was a milkman and she helped him with his horse-drawn deliveries three times a day. Even that image is hard to think of as having been just one generation prior to mine. The thing that I never really took on board was that when my mother was born, not all women in this country had the right to vote. Not until the Representation of the People (Equal Franchise) Act in 1928 were all adults over the age of twenty-one afforded suffrage, irrespective of sex or financial status. So I was the first in the matriarchal line to be born fully a 'person' in the eyes of the law. It had never occurred to me how that may have affected my hand-me-down sense of self. I needed to learn a little more about female suffrage.

Indulge me for a minute here with this quick catch-up on the female suffrage movement. It matters to our received sense of self, and it is important to take a moment to reflect on what we have internalised – laws may have changed, we may on paper be more equal as women than we ever have been, but it turns out that many of us are still reading from out-of-date scripts. It is widely accepted that democracy – *demokratia* (δημοκρατία, almost literally 'people power) – was first applied as a form of government in around 500BCE in Athens. However, even in those countries that call themselves democracies, governments are still working out who qualifies as a 'person'. Through my eyes it is taking far too long for humans to work out who *the people* are. For some time 'people' were exclusively male, usually white, persons with wealth and status; certainly slaves did not count among their number. And more than 2,500 years after the concept of democracy was born, women all over the world are still fighting to be recognised as full people.

In the late nineteenth century the battle for female suffrage began in many European and Commonwealth countries. It appeals to me that female descendants of *The Bounty* mutineers were the first women allowed to vote, on Pitcairn Island from 1838. In 1893, New Zealand became the first self-governing country to give the vote to all adult women, with Switzerland being the last in Europe to recognise women as full persons, giving them the vote in 1971. (The women of Switzerland's Appenzell canton were, however, not allowed to vote at cantonal level until 1990.)

Female suffrage movements have wrestled not only for the right to vote but also for the right to stand for election. Even when female suffrage was enacted, there were often no women to vote for. Women had to vote for men who would represent their interests. Often, the candidate was not concerned with empowering women; indeed it was likely in his interest to maintain the status quo. It remains the case that even where women have legal suffrage they often do not enjoy safe passage to cast their vote. Women's rights campaigners reported that in Zanzibar's 2015 general elections fifty women who voted were consequently divorced by their husbands for disobedience. In Uganda in 2016, many women were violently attacked for exercising their right of suffrage. It is hard to accept that, in the twenty-first century, women of the world are still not seen as full persons. I wondered if that was the case for me? Perhaps I wasn't as secure in my personhood as I thought? I had been very lucky in life. I felt secure in my role as a mother and as a professional woman, but in this new post-menopausal phase of my life did I no longer feel like a full person?

If the world still has a way to go in terms of female suffrage, it has even further to go to ensure women and girls feel safe from violence, particularly sexual violence. Many women I have spoken to, of all ages, are concerned for their personal safety – it affects almost every choice they make outside the home. Many do not feel safe to attend the theatre or concerts on their own after dark. And yet the truth is that women are most at risk in their own domestic spaces. Most European countries recognised spousal rape as a criminal offence in the late twentieth century, with the UK deeming it a sexual assault under the Sexual Offences Act as recently as 2003. Yet in 2018 the UK's *The Week* magazine reported that more than a third of people in Britain over the age of sixty-five do not regard forced marital sex to be rape. In February 2022, Smriti Irani, Minister for Women and Child Development in India, announced that the government was making provision for criminalising marital rape. The USA's journey towards protecting women from rape within a marriage, meanwhile, has been tortuous. The traditional definition of rape in North America is 'forced sexual intercourse by a male with a female not his wife' – which asks more questions than it answers, and has left each state to wrestle with its conscience. In 1986, during the era when my daughters were born, American feminist

Marie Shear remarked that 'Feminism is the radical notion that women are people.' My daughters are now mothers of daughters themselves. Come on world – change!

There is so much to be discussed about women's rights around the world: age of consent, definition of consent, domestic violence, abortion, access to contraception, and so on. However, that is not the focus of this book. So why do these issues matter in a book about Juicy Crones? They matter to every woman because they affect every single part of their life, from how safe they feel to the decisions they make. For the purpose of this book, it is useful to be mindful of how the issue of women's rights affects our sense of self. We cannot see ourselves as powerful, beautiful, wonderful, magical and 'free for the strangest adventures' if we are not even secure in the knowledge that we have the legal right to protection from sexual violence. For many women it is this fear that prevents them from going off and having adventures.

Set in the context of history, we are relatively new to seeing ourselves as equal, and millions of women around the world are still waiting for that day to dawn. It's easy to forget that women were not allowed a bank account in their own name in the UK until 1975. It was 1980 before we could apply for credit cards and loans, and 1982 before we could legally spend money in a pub.

In those countries where there is greater equality for all people, mainly in Scandinavia, everyone is happier – it is a net gain for everyone. One woman's gain is another man's – well, gain. Children certainly gain too. One is left wondering, why, oh why?

As I interviewed women for this book, it became clear that we were all processing conflicted feelings. Many of us had felt coerced by family and societal pressure into marrying in our early twenties and conforming to having children more or less immediately. Few of us had access to childcare and for the next twenty or more years we were occupied as wives and mothers, perhaps doing part-time work along the way. Some of us got our careers off the ground once the children were at school, but then came the double whammy of menopause, often while caring for ageing parents or partners became our priority. Of course we love and adore our children, and we want to care for family members, but those things come at great personal cost. It was not until post-menopause, with many still in caring roles, that we could lift our heads a little to survey the landscape. Many of the women I spoke to felt that it was only at this point, some forty or more years after their youth, that they realised they needed to take stock of what they had internalised. Their sense of self had, of course, absorbed cultural norms.

In the twentieth century, the mirror that was held up by society, the media and religion often reflected girls and women as smaller than life-sized – even those lucky enough to complete higher education. A woman needed to be small, dainty and quiet. She should be capable enough to be a suitable wife, but not too clever: she should never outshine her father or brothers or husband. She must give up her name on marriage and promise to 'obey' him. The mirror tells her she is not pretty enough – too fat, too thin, too pale, too dark. Her menstrual cycles should be coped with without fuss, and not be discussed or accommodated. She should marry young, have babies, and settle down quickly to be subordinate and to serve. She should hold the magic mirror for her husband and stroke him until he feels mighty enough to stride out; meanwhile, she must cut off bits of herself to make herself small enough to fit.

The Hall of Mirrors at the fair is sometimes funny, always confusing, and often frightening – everyone gets a distorted reflection. We often wish we could see ourselves as others do, but allowing ourselves the pain and challenge of seeing our true selves can be so rewarding. And this is not just true for women. Many men of a gentle nature were damaged by the historic expectations that they should go out and conquer, build castles and fiefdoms. Some men's egos were inflated to monstrous proportions, doing great harm to themselves, their families and wider society. Many girls grew up bitter, angry and unfulfilled. Many wives and mothers developed depression and a sense of self-loathing due to the tedium of day-to-day life and the physical contortions expected of them. Every one of us looking in a distorted mirror.

The mirroring from my childhood and adolescence went like this: my father was made the 'head of the household' by my mother, even though she was really the one with drive and ambition and the ability to be a leader. As a teenager during World War II, she worked in a bank in central London. A very clever woman, with impressive mental arithmetic skills, she soon became part of the mergers and acquisition team. As soon as the war ended, she had to relinquish her post to a returning soldier and found herself washing up in a café for a living. Once married, in many ways she was the puppet master: she washed, ironed and laid out my father's clothes, deciding for him what he should wear; she fed him his favourite foods, although after he died it turned out that many of these were actually *her* favourite foods. He was naturally a quiet man; she was naturally garrulous. She told us stories of *his* war. She pushed him to apply for promotion and celebrated his achievements with vicarious pride. She managed the family budget and worked hard to ensure that the head of the household delivered. No wonder, as in the fairground attraction, we were all confused; nothing was as it seemed. That is not to say that theirs was a bad marriage: we were happier and more loving than any other family I knew. It just wasn't an honest one. They both suffered because of societal pressures to conform to gender stereotypes. In all the households I knew as a child except one, male jobs were the important ones, the ones that had status and were protected at all costs. Disproportionate amounts of the household income went on ensuring that the men had clothes, food, alcohol and spare cash for hobbies – including gambling. Wives stroked and flattered them, and children were expected to wait on them. They took their place at the head of the table. They drove the car. The household often revolved around upholding the status of the father. At work, almost all bosses were male and almost all men earned more than women, even for the same work.

Generally speaking, I didn't experience a great deal of sexism throughout my working life. The world of education, social care and health, the three arenas I worked in, were predominantly female. I was used to female bosses – indeed I was one. Women's voices were heard, and drove policy and practice. My specialisms, educating young minds, and later children's health and well-being, were comfortably 'female'. What I did not realise until I left work was that I had not integrated the strengths and qualities of my work persona into my personal identity. I had viewed myself as an independent, successful woman, yet as soon as I retired I realised this was a veneer beneath which existed a flimsy sense of self. The two were separate in my mind, which might account in part for why I found retirement distressing: I simply did not recognise myself.

Retirement presented me with a personal, existential crisis. The loss of my sense of self revealed some very painful truths to me. We all have a box of metaphorical masks or hats that we wear when the situation requires us to. Like everyone else, I had a large basketful which I had drawn upon, as and when needed, at different times in my life: the good little girl, the self-sacrificing wife, the caring teacher, the professional woman with matching suits, the Mummy, the caring daughter. I'm not suggesting these were false fronts, but they were relational and often focused on meeting the needs of others. Some of these masks I chose to remove – by retiring, certainly, and when reluctantly accepting that my children were now grown and had flown the nest. Others were painful to remove: when my parents died and I would no longer be anyone's daughter and, in the natural order of things, would be the next generation to go – easy to say, but much harder to accept. Long years of mourning followed, in which I worked though my loss, sorrow and regret.

Gradually, over the course of many months, it dawned on me that removing the masks or hats I had worn for so long was not the biggest challenge: it was the loss of my sense of self when I was not behind them. I had embodied my masks just as, when I was growing up, I had embodied misogyny and homophobia. I had allowed them to silence the real me.

I slowly came to realise that my self-confidence, my sense of accomplishment, my happiness, my status in the world, all felt uncertain, and that each time I removed one of my masks my purpose was being torn away. It seemed that the veneer that remained was worryingly thin and susceptible to being ripped or lost altogether.

It was in this rather fragile and vulnerable state that I started to find meaning and purpose in retirement. It is no wonder that, with one or two exceptions, I found my journey to be a rutted and rain-soaked one. Nothing felt like it quite fitted.

I began to see that, despite the odds stacked against me, I had been remarkably determined and resilient. I had always felt I was fighting something, going against the flow, shoulder to the wheel. Life for me had been a herculean task, always striving, always feeling that I had to do more, to prove myself, to earn my place in the world, seeking approval and love wherever I went.

Understanding what processes had made 'me' is an ongoing labour – peeling back those layers is not for the faint-hearted. True *knowing* is experiential, about feeling, not academic understanding.

Lamination is a layering process which occurs in the natural world; in geology, for example. (It is also one of the highlights of the *Great British Bake Off* competition, when contestants try to get as many layers as possible into their bread or pastry.) In industry, lamination is applied to give strength, stability and structure. The concept is simple: one thin layer is placed on top of another and glued together with adhesive. Almost imperceptibly, the layers grow into a what at first glance can look like a single solid structure. The layers are heated above their melting point until they are bonded together. Often, huge amounts of rolling pressure are brought to bear on the lamination over time, to merge the materials and ensure compliance to the form required.

While lamination can produce immensely strong structures, once something starts to delaminate it can crack, buckle, corrode or totally collapse – as is sometimes seen on bridges and piers. Delamination can be catastrophic. Sometimes the structure is beyond repair and has to be rebuilt from scratch.

That is how this part of my life felt – as if it was delaminating in a dramatic and seemingly catastrophic way. I didn't know how to stop the layers falling apart, twisting, separating. The previous few years had been corrosive, eating away at my happiness and contentment. The edges were splintered, I had lost my strength and flexibility, and – worse still – I didn't know where to begin making repairs. I didn't know myself. The form and the textures were unfamiliar and unreliable. The only way was through. I sought help in various forms of psychotherapy and will always be grateful to those who supported me through the rollercoaster ride. I sometimes felt that I was being torn apart, mainly because I was impatient to get to the bottom of it.

With the benefit of hindsight, I can see that what had happened to me and millions of other women was akin to being brainwashed into a cult, or radicalisation. It was in many ways a structurally cruel world. During the brainwashing process the subject's identity is broken down until their identity falls apart. It can then be replaced by a set of behaviours, attitudes and beliefs that serve the needs of the cult. Which of us hasn't felt obliged to take someone else's name on marriage, hasn't bristled at only being referred to as 'Jo's mummy', hasn't thought we had to accept surviving on three hours sleep a night for several years, or felt overwhelmed trying to homeschool during a global pandemic while working from home – because women are good at multitasking, aren't they?

There is much debate about whether brainwashing is effective. Most of the women I have met didn't really *believe* they were less than, they didn't really *believe* they should have to use someone else's name, they didn't really *believe* they should be defined by how they looked. But the weight of coercion was so great, or their opportunity to make other choices so few, that they felt the only option was to comply. You were the daughter of a man until he 'gave you away' – and then you became the wife of a man. Fundamentally, our layers had been heated to above melting point and there was no possibility but to bow to their weight.

But compliance doesn't stop anger and resentment fermenting inside. It's no wonder that, statistically, women in the UK experience more mental health issues than men. We've been subjected to injustice for so long we have reason to be mad.

Much of the lamination that my generation of women experienced was toxic. Girlfriends of mine at the secondary modern school I was condemned to were made to leave school to help on the farm, or earn money in a shop, before they had a chance to sit examinations, severely limiting their life chances. The appearance of legislation such as the right to abortion in 1963, the Equal Pay Act in 1974 and the availability of the pill during the 1960s served only to distort our understanding further. Despite these advances, we were still not paid equally (and still are not) and were still expected to put our careers on hold or give them up to have a family. The sexual revolution often made women feel as if they should be more 'available' to men rather than helping them understand their own sexual needs. The very British phenomenon of the 'Page 3 girl' only served to confuse and anger further. For some it was a sign of progressiveness, for others it represented exploitation and coercive control.

I had extra layers of lamination brainwashed into me by the Christian fundamentalism of the chapel that my parents belonged to. I learned that I was born sinful and that I would go to hell unless I met unattainable standards of moral behaviour. My body was a temple of the holy spirit and not mine to do with as I wanted. Most sensible children rejected this as a load of hooey as soon as they heard it. Unfortunately for me, I was a dutiful, sensitive child who absorbed everything I was told.

The chapel was governed and controlled by the elders, who were all self-appointed men. Women were not allowed to speak in chapel, either to read aloud from the Bible or to deliver the sermon, although they could teach in the Sunday School and play the harmonium if the male organist was absent. They had to follow St Paul's teaching to cover their heads, to ensure they were not detracting from the glory of God, and were required to wear 'Sunday best' to chapel, which should reveal nothing above the knee, nor their arms (and trousers were not permitted). They were also expected to volunteer to clean the church, arrange flowers and make cakes for events. In the outside world most families read the *News of the World* and *Titbits*, and watched *Carry On* films and the Miss World contest. Each week we watched Morecambe and Wise sharing a bed and no-one said a word. It was no wonder I was confused.

Almost every woman I have spoken to while researching this book has struggled to put herself first – and has seen meeting her own needs as selfish. This misplaced guilt prevents women from leading the post-menopausal life they want. What seems to be common is that, like trauma victims, women often don't know what they need – they don't know when they are tired, hungry, satiated. They may not recognise or accept emotions such as anger, jealousy or even pride, thereby erasing part of who they truly are. Perhaps this is because many women have been lifelong carers and have put the needs of others first for so long that they have learned to deny their own feelings, and even their bodily needs.

Every woman in this book, including me, has journeyed through a 'dark night of the soul'. Mostly they travelled alone because they assumed, wrongly, that this was uniquely their problem. They may have sought medical help, for which the solution proffered was very likely antidepressants, or heard a well-meaning friend telling them to 'count their blessings'. However, few would admit to feeling that the post-menopausal age was a personal existential crisis that needed more than an Elastoplast to heal.

During menopause, the façades we adopt can start to buckle and peel like some water-soaked kitchen work surface. But this delamination, however painful, opens up choices about how we reconstruct ourselves. What do we want now as meaning and purpose in our life, and how will we be proactive in our choosing?

I wish for all of us to belt out with my granddaughters: 'We are powerful, beautiful, wonderful, magical and FREE. Oh, and by the way, we are not our mistakes.'

3

ARIADNE'S THREAD

It's not enough for us to merely observe the scope of the problems women face in our modern medical system or even to voice our feelings of anger and betrayal at what we see; we need to be always asking, 'What can we do about this?'

Dr Alyson J McGregor, *Sex Matters*

For many years I taught in a girls' school. I was head of years 8 and 9 (12–14 years old) and I taught religious studies, philosophy and ethics. I was also head of personal, social and health education (PSHE). The latter was seen as a Cinderella subject, but I never felt like that about it. I always believed that it offered some of the most important time the girls spent, time for thinking about their own health and well-being, time to discuss these subjects with their friends – and a place to get reliable information about sensitive subjects. It provided a pause in the week, relief from the pressure of academic achievement and a slight challenge to the myth that everything important had to be examined and recognised with a certificate. This was about empowerment: teaching them how to think and how to keep themselves physically and mentally well.

My main aim was to provide the girls with the most up-to-date information about mental health, self-harm, grooming, consent, drugs, alcohol, sex, pregnancy, sexually transmitted diseases – the curriculum was as wide and varied as the needs of the girls I taught. It was important too, that the girls had the space to think about the ethical impacts of their choices. So, for example, drug education needed a global perspective. Seeing the international drug business in its entirety – from the drug lords in Colombia through the drug mules distributing the product, from the hundreds of exploited and vulnerable teenagers groomed for county-line work to the sex workers in the street, often working to support an addiction or lured into prostitution by dealers – gave them insight into what they were supporting if they bought a bag of cocaine at a party. In the same way, by looking at the global textile industry, and the seemingly simple act of buying a pair of jeans in our local supermarket, we opened a window on to our personal responsibility around chemical pollution, deforestation and threats to indigenous people.

After retirement, I spent many years trying to find my way to a place of recognition of self. As in the myth of Ariadne's thread, I needed to find my way by exhausting all routes and moving through the labyrinths to understanding. I was trying to inform myself about what I needed to know to be as healthy, in every sense of the word, as I could. There's an adage that we teach in order to understand. And maybe we need to understand in order to teach. I've come to realise that if I were teaching PSHE to the girls now, I would take a somewhat different stance. It would be their human rights that I'd want to emphasise, just as much as those of the drug workers and the indigenous peoples of the world. So prevalent is the discrimination and indifference to the needs of women's health, it is staggering and shocking beyond anything that a drug overlord may be doing from atop his eyrie.

In the couple of years since I started writing this book, my local bookshop has been filling up with more and more books written by well-educated, entertaining and erudite women – leaders in their chosen field. Thank heavens for that. It is like a breath of fresh air to be able to read about the things I need to know about. I think particularly of Caroline Criado Perez's *Invisible Women*, Lisa Mosconi's *The XX Brain*, Mary Ann Sieghart's *The Authority Gap*, Dr Alyson McGregor's *Sex Matters* and Naomi Wolf's *Vagina*, all of which shine a light on the specific needs of women and how, often, these needs are not currently being met. We *are* learning more, but that is just exposing how little we knew, how badly served we have been over many centuries by traditional medicine, and how low down the priority list we are. It is no wonder that so many women turn (and this is often sneered at) to alternative or complementary medicine. Perhaps that's because women have found help there, and discovered that their bodies can tolerate the medicine, or supplements as they must by law be known.

I would advise the girls now that, should their GP recommend a prescription drug, they ask: 'Has it been tested on women? And if it has been tested on women, were the results disaggregated?' That is, were the findings of the study separated into male and female? Criado Perez in *Invisible Women* walks us through the gender data gap, revealing how few medicines have been trialled on women and, where they have, how rarely we are informed about the side effects, good or bad, that women experience. How many of us have had unpleasant or frightening side effects from a prescription drug, not realising that perhaps it might be because the drug has not been trialled on women – and that we are effectively the unsupervised guinea pig.

Largely because our hormone fluctuations have traditionally been seen as inconvenient, and introduce too many variables into trial situations, it is only relatively recently that women have been included in drug trials. Now that such information may be available to us, it's important to know if the effects and side effects of drugs differ for women and men. Asking your doctor if a drug has been trialled on women may well annoy them, and they probably won't immediately know the answer – but a good GP will, hopefully, say, 'I'll find out for you.' The point is that, if we keep asking the questions, we will exert pressure for change. Rarely do men need to ask their GP, 'Was this drug tested on men?' The very question sounds silly. As Janette (page 146) quipped when we discussed this – we need a sticker, as for 'Not Tested on Animals', with the Rabbit logo, saying 'Not Tested on Women'. (Which symbol would be apt, I wonder?) We are in an age that is moving towards personalised medicine, which is in itself very exciting, but in the meantime there is power in knowledge and we all need access to the most up-to-date information available.

In *Sex Matters*, Dr Alyson McGregor retells how her choice of women's health as a specialism in the early 2000s was assumed to focus on reproductive medicine – commonly called 'bikini medicine'. Women were seen as the same as men, but with 'boobs and tubes'. But in reality she was interested in the *whole* woman – female chromosomes exist in every cell of our bodies, they affect the way our bodies develop, they impact on every disease and therefore the way in which we should be treated. Dr McGregor also co-founded the Sex and Gender Women's Health Collaborative, working to improve knowledge and understanding of the importance of including sex as a biological variable in research design.

Up until very recently, medical textbooks were illustrated with only the male form. Occasional 'out-boxes' were sometimes added to illustrate the female reproductive system. Like the Shetland Isles to the rest of the UK, or Socotra to Yemen: interesting and alluring, but not mainland. The first comprehensive anatomical study of the clitoris was led by the urologist Professor Helen O'Connell and published in 1998. Just read that sentence again: there is a part of the female body (and there are others) that until a couple of decades ago had never been the subject of rigorous anatomical study. I'm trying not to be a cynic, but it's hard not to wonder if that's because the main function of the clitoris is pleasure – enjoying our body? In the twenty-five years since Professor O'Connell's study, this knowledge, the fact that the main function of the clitoris is pleasure, remains largely absent from the medical curriculum. If you are starting to feel that this is the kind of book you wouldn't want your mother to catch you reading, that's the point. Somehow, somewhere along the line we have learned to feel awkward or embarrassed when it comes to understanding our own bodies – they can often feel like forbidden territory, even though they belong to us! While we are encouraged to look after our health, to love our bodies, that's quite hard to do when so little money has gone into researching women's health. It is difficult to be informed because either we don't appear in studies or our doctors, half of whom are now female, have not always been trained in women's health needs and anatomy. Despite being more than fifty per cent of the population, we are still often seen as 'outliers'. We can only hope that future generations of doctors are better educated.

Back to my students. They need to know that if they are one of the ten per cent or more of women who develop endometriosis, much of the time they will be fobbed off by doctors or told they are imagining it. On average it will take seven years to get a diagnosis and those years can be hell. I would also tell the girls that most, around eighty per cent, of them are likely to suffer from premenstrual syndrome (PMS). That might take the form of some discomfort that requires pain relief, but it might also be so severe that they will end up in agony, curled up in bed or throwing up, utterly depressed. It may make them feel like they can't eat for a week, or conversely that all they want to do is to eat crisps and chocolate. They may be so moody that they can't get along with themselves. And I would warn them that they may be disbelieved, or their pain minimised.

In more optimistic news, the journalist Ida Emilie Steinmark reported in April 2022 in *The Guardian* newspaper some hope for new treatments for painful and heavy periods. According to Steinmark, menstruation is to be wondered at – biologically speaking the process is odd, and the majority of animals don't do it. We are apparently closest, in matters menstrual, to spiny mice. What I find strange is that funding for research has been so low; that we know so little about something that happens to women every month for around forty years of their life. We don't even know what is 'normal'. There have been no new treatments for the associated pain and heavy bleeding for thirty years. Thirty years!

In *Invisible Women*, Criado Perez notes that PMS is chronically understudied and that attempts to get funding for research are often met with denial of the condition's existence. She cites a 2013 study of sildenafil citrate, which gave total relief of PMS symptoms with no side effects. Sildenafil had been trialled in the early 1990s for heart disease. That trial was made up entirely of male subjects and had a surprising outcome: the development of a drug now most widely known as Viagra. Ker-ching! As Criado Perez says, 'a happy ending for men, then'.

Health education needs to arm girls and women to shoot back the arrows of gaslighting. They need to be forewarned that even the language used to describe their anatomy has an agenda; they may be described, like me, as being in a state of atrophy, as having an 'incompetent' cervix, 'inhospitable' womb, 'irritable' uterus, 'poor' ovarian reserve or a womb 'incompatible' with life. They may exert 'poor' maternal effort, or be 'barren'. One woman, speaking on BBC Radio 4's *Woman's Hour*, told of how, after suffering the agony of stillbirth, her unborn baby was described to her as 'naughty' for not behaving as it should in utero. I can't think of any medical terminology used of men that is judgemental in this way.

It seems that conventional medicine has ingested the belief that women are 'hysterical' in mind and body. Women need to just 'calm down, dear'. Every woman I have spoken to has been offered antidepressants for whatever they present at their family doctor, be it menopause, migraine or post-viral fatigue. It's the modern-day equivalent of leeching.

I would want the girls to trust themselves to know that they have real symptoms, real pain and the right to treatment that is suited to their needs as women. I winced when I heard Sajid Javid, the UK's Health Secretary at the time, state that doctors too often ignore women's pain. He was right, and I am grateful that he made a stand, but it's unbelievable that it needed to be said in the twenty-first century. Many societies, especially those that hold to the Genesis story, have embodied the belief that women deserve to experience pain, since Eve was responsible for the corruption of Adam at 'the Fall'. We corrupted man and therefore deserve to be punished. Even today women are expected to undergo painful gynaecological procedures without effective pain relief.

It turns out then, my focus should have been on teaching the girls which questions to ask of mainstream medicine to empower them to receive better healthcare. Yes, there's still a place for education about illegal drugs. But the mythical drug dealer at the school gate is, perhaps, less of a danger to them than not being in receipt of the facts – the medical education needed to serve them as informed women.

Like me, I doubt my fellow Juicy Crones had any health education at school. What little I knew I got from the back pages of my mother's *My Weekly*. I was shocked by my own lack of medical knowledge when I read Naomi Wolf's book *Vagina* (I think she had been shocked about her own lack of medical knowledge, too). How could it be that I had got to my mid-sixties and not know these things? I had spent my whole adult life in health education and am unembarrassed talking about sex, bodies or, indeed, feelings, but I had never, for example, seen medical diagrams of the anatomy of the female pelvic nerves, which varies greatly from those of males. There was so much for me yet to learn about my own body.

As I've already touched upon, another area sorely lacking in information is the menopause. In 2021, Diane Danzebrink, founder of the #MakeMenopauseMatter campaign, put a Freedom of Information request to the UK's thirty-three medical schools asking if menopause was on their curriculum for doctors in training. Shockingly, only forty-one per cent of those schools replied in the affirmative. So, at the time of writing, the UK's thirteen million perimenopausal and menopausal women are likely to visit a doctor who has had no formal training in the menopause or hormone replacement therapy.

Dr Louise Newson, a GP and menopause specialist, has done extraordinary work trying to redress the lack of menopause education and training for health professionals by offering free online training for all healthcare workers anywhere in the world.

There are private clinics springing up that offer consultations and bespoke regimens for menopausal women. But for many women the cost is prohibitive. High-profile campaigners such as Mariella Frostrup and Davina McCall have moved us forward a great deal in terms of menopause being talked about in the public domain, but there is still a long way to go.

It's not just in the area of reproductive systems that women differ so widely from men. Dr Lisa Mosconi in *The XX Brain* aims to empower women to prevent dementia. She highlights that women's brains age differently from men's and that we need to take care of ourselves in our wisdom years to keep ourselves well. We are at greater risk of developing dementia than breast cancer and two-thirds of Alzheimer's patients are female. The right to information and treatment that would protect our long-term brain health is key. Mosconi outlines the ways in which we can mitigate this frightening increased risk, from receiving the right hormone replacement therapy, to taking care over environmental toxins, to being more socially active, ensuring that we make our neurons fire in new ways, to the importance of oral hygiene – early evidence is emerging of a connection between periodontal disease and brain inflammation. We also need to know how to keep our bones strong to protect against osteoporosis, that signs of a heart attack present differently in women – and how we can articulate that to the medical profession.

Why does all this matter, you ask – isn't this book about older women going off and having adventures? Well, yes, that's a fair question, but the point is that for us all to stay well and active for as long as possible we need to know how to best take care of our health. Those women, and there are many, with health issues getting in the way of them leading the life they want, need to have access to the right medical care and attention in order to support their ambitions – whether that's climbing Kilimanjaro, passing the medical for a pilot licence or relaxing in the garden.

If you ever doubt the importance of public health information, just reflect on what we all learned during the Covid pandemic. We all now have it within our grasp to read graphs, spot trends, assess our personal risk and take the best course of action armed with the most up-to-date information. We all know how to prevent infectious diseases spreading and we know how to take a swab from our nose and throats. We have seen that it is possible to be well informed, to take responsibility for our health and to improve our chances of leading a long, healthy and fulfilling life.

Had I been able to access the kind of advice, treatment and support now offered by Dr Louise Newson and others, ten or more years of my life may have been quite different. I went to my doctor to discuss distressing menopausal symptoms, but I was advised against HRT because of my history of breast cysts and my family history of breast cancer. I will never know how much of these gruelling ten years was due to post-viral fatigue and how much was a tricky menopause. My suspicion is that it was a diabolical combination of the two. All I know is that I lost a decade of my life to feeling unwell, living a foggy and fragmented life.

To my great joy, many of the extraordinary young women I used to teach went on to become doctors, midwives and other health professionals. I would hope they are shaking up the systems as they go through, questioning outmoded ways of thinking and providing the best available healthcare for women.

4

REACHING SCRATCH

One must start from scratch – and it takes a very long time to reach scratch.

Philosopher Elizabeth Anscombe, speaking to her friend
Iris Murdoch, as quoted in *Metaphysical Animals* by
Clare Mac Cumhaill and Rachael Wiseman

Elizabeth Anscombe was referring to philosophy when she spoke these words, but the more I sought understanding from my fellow crones, the more apt it felt in relation to post-menopausal life.

Theoretically it's hard to imagine why I didn't just step off the platform of my career and step on to the train to a fulfilling retirement. I'd been a successful woman at work; I'd been, I hope, a good enough mother, and a dutiful, loving daughter. Why wasn't I stepping forward with self-confidence, excitement and courage? I think it was about role models – I knew what a successful manager looked like, I knew what kind of mother I was aspiring to be, but when it came to putting on the mantle of 'retired woman', first of all I hadn't given it a moment's thought, but when I did, I realised that, apart from my mother, I hardly knew any older women. That is, I hadn't had conversations that got beneath the skin of what it was *really* like to be post-menopausal. There were plenty in the media who I admired, but few in my own life who I could aspire to be like. What kind of crone was I or did I want to be? Where did she hang out? What did she wear? Where did she go to have fun? Where did her sense of self, her identity, come from? I could only answer this question by feeling my way through.

Putting pen to paper here demands that I give chronology and structure to events. But only with hindsight do my baby steps into this phase of my life feel like they had any kind of order to them. Trust me, it did not feel planned at all in the lived experience. While it was happening, it felt completely random, as if I were flailing around in a truly unglamorous fashion, more bagatelle than bowls.

Luckily for me, I journaled more or less daily throughout this time. Journaling was a conscious effort to keep hold of my sanity, which at times felt perilously close to unravelling. My sense of self was so fragile that it sometimes felt like I was disappearing altogether. Could I give myself permission to find out who I was, even if I didn't like what I found?

For me and many other women I have spoken to, post-menopause can feel chaotic. So, whereas I would like to say if you do X followed by Y, then Z will follow, I can't. This is not a self-help book and one size never does fit all. Rather like painting in pre-school, the post-menopausal age is messy and wild, the apron never quite covers it and … it takes ages to clear up. But it can be bright, exciting and fun, and you get lots to show for it. Hopefully, you'll emerge feeling energised, stronger and in touch with the authentic you – whatever that entails. To paraphrase the artist Paul Klee, you must adapt to the contents of your paintbox. Few women of my generation have the resources to fund an ascent of K9 or a month's retreat on Dartmoor. However, many have given themselves the gift of venturing into the wild for free or have discovered the joy of living simply in nature.

There is no destination when it comes to being a Juicy Crone. This is a time to ignore all those magazines hectoring us to weigh and measure ourselves, to judge our performance in life – even the ones aimed at mental health can make us feel as if we *should* be meditating better or *improving* our mindfulness – just adding to our anxiety and hypervigilance. This is a time to do it our way. This journey is about finding a way to self, to peace and contentment, whether that is single-handedly sailing the Pacific, painting with mud, or enjoying some radical rest – the sheer joy of doing *nothing* should never be undervalued.

Received wisdom has it that post-menopause is a place to wither and die (if you could just finish the ironing first). Which brings us back to atrophy again – the default image of the older woman in our society. Men wither too, but no-one cares. It doesn't even warrant comment. No-one says of David Attenborough: doesn't white hair age him? Without realising it, I had ingested beliefs about what it means to be an older woman and, as is often the case, it was paradoxical. We could expect a steady decline of mind and body – wrinkles, arthritis, memory loss and sagging everything – and yet we needed to 'look young', not have grey hair, continue with caring responsibilities, often with very limited resources. In my case the chronic fatigue and 'atrophy' diagnosis had compounded this, but I needed to work out where my thinking was flawed. I needed to give myself permission to learn who I was at this stage in my life. So, while physicians and the world seemed to see me in decline, if not invisible, I slowly started to experience this as a joyful emergence, a reawakening.

What follows is a telling of my personal odyssey to make sense of this part of my life. Like Odysseus I faced many storms and shipwrecks along the way. It's one thing having the 'wake-up' call, that yes, you are in your third act – but quite another knowing what it is saying. There were tears and tantrums and moments of elation. I felt old and achy, young and energised; witchy and wizened, playful and sassy. It was a unique experience, but in some ways similar to how I felt in my teenage years. I was trying things on for size to see what fitted, to discover what felt like *me* and what didn't.

In our heads many of us are still about nineteen or thereabouts – about to grab life… and then life grabs us. On that first day, in the ground zero of my post-retirement life, I was under no illusion. I was one of the very lucky ones. I was in goodish health, despite the post-viral fatigue, I was financially comfortable, I lived in a place I loved and had a wonderful family. You might well think, how very lucky is she – what else did she want? And that would be a fair criticism. It wasn't a matter of having the 'I wants', though. I had no desire or need for material things. What I was seeking was meaning and purpose. Equally, I was aware of my tendency to jump into everything with both feet and then end up being chairperson of this, or leader of that. I did have the wisdom at that point to give myself time for reflection, a sabbatical if you like, to ponder before I took on any new responsibilities.

Some habits are impossible to break. Waking very early was mine. One of the seemingly banal first treats I indulged in was the deep joy to be found in having a tray of tea in bed and greeting each dawn with journaling, reading or just, well, just being. In all my days since, throughout my search for what it means to be juicy, that pleasure has endured as a daily indulgence and is often my most creative time.

Stepping into retirement I was very aware of the negative connotations. Even the word retire – leave, step down, cease, retreat, withdraw – was hard to spin. Perhaps because I had had several years of ill health, it was impossible to ignore the large EXIT sign looming; but statistically speaking, if I was very lucky, I could have many active years left.

At one of the last presentations I gave at work, for the launch of an initiative to support and improve the mental health of children and young people, a delegate asked how I would measure its success. I remember my answer: when we no longer differentiate between physical and mental health, neither one being more important nor better funded than the other – when we see health as a holistic entity. I knew that if I was to have a happy, healthy retirement, I needed to look after myself holistically. Mind, body, soul. What was it that made me feel alive? Where would I find my bliss? It was surprising to discover when I answered myself honestly just how much of my thinking was directed by 'should' or 'ought'.

I had spent many years focusing on the health of children and young people and writing endless strategic plans with actions and achievable outcomes. Surely, I should be able to write a strategic plan for my own well-being. The problem was, well, that I didn't really know what the problem was, and I didn't know what I was trying to achieve apart from that elusive concept of happiness. Happiness isn't a destination, it's a by-product, the feeling we get when we are in 'flow', or 'doing our thing'. I needed to find my flow. Where would I find it? And how? Only, it turned out, by trial and error.

I'd retired in January, my partner was still in full-time work, my health was improving, but I was a way off being fully well. I wanted to mark this time with a long, but manageable, walk. I took an hour's flight from Bristol to Guernsey and booked a week in a bed and breakfast in St Peter Port. It's a very manageable four-day walk around the island – mostly easy underfoot with a few strenuous ups and downs on the south coast. Guernsey has a very good bus service, which meant that I could base myself in St Peter Port and pick up the route where I left off the day before. It also provided a safety net – if the coast path got too much (it didn't), I could walk up to the road and wait for a bus. I learned a lot about myself that week. I was incredibly lucky to have glorious, crisp winter sunshine. In the middle of one day I lay down high on a grassy knoll and realised that I had overridden my needs for so long that I didn't know when I was tired, or hungry or thirsty. Did I know what I was really feeling? It was as basic as that – I needed to tune in to myself if I was to take better care of me. Sylvia Plath's words in *The Bell Jar* came to me: '*I* wasn't *steering* anything, not even *myself*.'

My few days on Guernsey served as the opening of a new chapter. It was a beginning, a slight easing of the disconnect I felt and a positive experience from which to continue my journey.

In late spring, I went back to my village, my river, my school on Salisbury Plain. I felt it was important in my quest to understand what had made me – how was my sense of self formed? To my relief, my river had not changed at all. I could walk across the same broken bridges, see the horses' hoofmarks in the small patch of tatty tarmac, sit on the creamy-chalky bank and watch the fish jumping where we used to scramble in to swim. I didn't see a kingfisher that day but felt confident that I might. I was still mesmerised by the curtains of green-black weed sweeping and shimmering across the gleaming white river bottom, fish sweeping and shimmering in unison. It recaptured my deep love of this place, lit with a gentle sun, screened by overhanging willows and reeds.

I walked southwards across the flower-rich grassland from my village of Durrington Walls towards the playground of my childhood, skylarks trilling overhead. The River Avon, hidden in the trees below, where I spent so many hours playing as a child, has an important historical role in marking the ritual of human passing. It is thought that early humans brought their loved ones here to their final resting place, via the river and Woodhenge and on to the cursus of Stonehenge, that early cathedral of mystery and awe. Stonehenge pays homage to the wonder that is our natural world, aligning humankind with the stars and moon and marking their place within nature. I felt immensely grateful that in the great lottery of birth, I opened my eyes so very near here, in a village in the middle of Salisbury Plain. I felt completely connected to the chalky earth, to the vast open skies and to the absolute luxury of the freedom to roam. Those feelings had always spelled home for me. Now, sixty years later, I could return and have them flood through me once more. Part of learning who I am has been to embrace my need to connect with that essence of unfettered wandering. Whatever aspects of myself were 'add-ons', this was not one of them – this was the core of me.

Not all my journeys were so literal. One of the things I fancied doing was to learn to draw. In fact, any kind of art appealed. I had been hopeless at school, but then we were not 'taught' art at all – you were somehow expected to just know how to do it. A local watercolour course caught my eye, and I was tempted until I saw it was held in the craft room of the local nursing home. That really was a bridge too far for me. So, I signed up for 'Drawing for the Terrified' at the nearby Nature in Art Museum. This was what I needed – a step-by-step guide on how to look, hold a pencil, develop an eye for shape and colour, blend colours. Basic steps. It was so satisfying and helped me make friends with being a beginner.

For so long I had needed to be an authority in my area of expertise – now here I was knowing nothing. The more things I tried, the more I found this 'beginner's mind' liberating. I took instruction and gave it my best shot. 'Beginner's mind', or *shoshin*, is a word from Zen Buddhism. At the time of my baby steps into this new world of retirement I didn't know of its existence. But now I experienced for myself the freedom in focusing excitement and energy towards something new. With an open mind and no preconceptions, anything was possible. It relieved me of the shame-based feelings of not being 'good enough'. It was OK, in fact better, to not know anything. I knew nothing, so there were no rights or wrongs, just me having fun exploring. Like a kid wandering around Salisbury Plain again. I tried hard to vanquish the chattering voices in my head, full of criticism. In her book *This Too Shall Pass*, psychotherapist Julia Samuel calls these her 'shitty committee', which always makes me smile. I try to replace them with kinder voices marvelling at the joy of new experiences. New ways of seeing are refreshing and liberating.

I then went on a weekend drawing course. The aim was to come to drawing 'new' (which in my case wasn't hard). We drew with our non-dominant hand, with our eyes closed, we drew smells and sounds, anything to shake us out of our preconceptions. I loved it; it suited my brain entirely and I brushed off some of the chips on my shoulder about 'being rubbish at art'. It no longer mattered – I was having fun. In fact, some of the pieces I did with my left hand I kept. Something about me had been portrayed there – I didn't know what, but I knew it was significant!

It became clear that I needed to give myself permission to have fun and just enjoy life. What? I attended another day course, this one called 'Selfish' with life coach Theresa Sansome. All the delegates were female, and all of us held the concept that to do anything for ourselves was *selfish*. That everything, especially if we did it alone or it cost money, had to be either utilitarian or in some other way justifiable.

People can get rather sneery about this experimentation: 'Oh, she's trying to *reinvent* herself.' I wasn't trying to reinvent anything. I was trying to uncover aspects of self that had been long submerged or talents that I had never had time to develop. Small children can do everything – sing, dance, paint, draw, tell stories – until gradually their talents are corralled and they become defined as 'good at maths', 'sporty' or 'poor at art'. I found this time wonderfully freeing, just as my life had been before formal education started.

Amid all these new activities, I had started to scribble – jottings in a journal, in many ways reminiscent of the indulgent outpourings of teenage angst. I suppose the similarities were no coincidence – I was in the middle of a major life transition and there was no guidebook to help me navigate. There were a few self-help books about life over fifty, but they weren't addressing the things I was trying to find answers to. They offered practical hints and tips on finances and fashion, beauty and fitness, but didn't help me find the inspiration I needed.

My scribbling became a routine part of my morning tea ritual. I looked around for writing workshops. I found an intriguing one at Hawkwood College in Stroud, an evening course in 'Wild Writing'. Now you're talking! That sounded like me. The tutor, a modern-day bard, was terrific and understood that I was a beginner. We responded to his prompts, wrote for five minutes, and then listened to each other's pieces. It was my first experience of reading my writing out loud and of being a critical friend to others. A small spark was lit in me. I attended a few other workshops and began to write almost obsessively. In part this was writing as therapy, getting my thoughts and feelings about the past on to paper, to help make sense of my life. Largely it felt like I was writing myself back into my own story. I started to write without any censorship – exactly how I felt, being as honest as I could with myself about my thoughts and feelings. This was an entirely private matter. It was sometimes painful to face my own truth, but cathartic and enabling.

I continued to walk as much and as often as I could, which for me was the best healing for both mind and body. Gradually, as I got my physical strength back, I started to build up stamina in the local swimming pool and challenged myself by walking in the Malvern Hills. I had done plenty of hill walking as a young woman and I experienced again how by gaining physical height we can gain emotional perspective too. We become dots on a hillside and get a wide-angle view of the landscape. Progress was slow and incremental, but enough that I could feel myself getting stronger. More importantly I began to feel the joy of it.

The opportunity came for me to do a sponsored walk across Morecambe Bay in aid of the RNLI. The metaphors here, of quicksink and rescue boats, are irresistible. The walk offered the promise of a personal challenge and a way to understand a little more about why I often felt as if I were standing on sinking sands – as well, of course, as raising money for this wonderful organisation.

The sands of Morecambe Bay are some of the most treacherous in the world. Many people have lost their lives attempting to walk across – or even just play on – them. In 2004, more than twenty Chinese cockle pickers, being paid a pittance, lost their lives two and a half miles out from Bolton-le-Sands. It's a huge tidal bay, sometimes known as the wet Sahara, and the sands move dramatically with every incoming and outgoing tide. The rivers Lune, Keer, Wyre and Leven all flow out into the bay, opening up new river channels as each tide retreats – which can be as much as seven miles – while, because the bay is so flat, the returning waters roar in at up to ten knots, rising up to thirty-two feet deep, and taking no prisoners. Tractors, transit vans and horses have disappeared without trace within seconds.

I spent four years as a student in this area. One of the reasons I chose Lancaster University as an undergraduate was its proximity to the Lake District and the fine walking to be had there. Indeed, I spent almost every weekend of my years at Lancaster walking in the lakes and dales. In my second year I lived in a student flat in Morecambe, which, rather unkindly, was known in winter as a 'cemetery with lights'. The winter of 1977 was particularly ferocious. West End Pier was besieged by a storm, and friends with basement flats lost everything, including their handwritten dissertations, as the sea filled their rooms to the ceiling.

This was an area well known to me, and the sponsored walk became part of my quest to understand myself – to return to that place and integrate the events of those years, good and bad. The walk, eight miles across wet sand from Arnside to Grange-over-Sands, was led by Cedric Robinson, the Queen's Guide to the Sands. There has been a Royal Guide to the Sands since the 1500s, when to walk this way had the advantage of avoiding a very lengthy and poorly maintained coastal road. About halfway across there is a waist-deep crossing through the channel of the River Kent. It was going to be a huge challenge for me, both physically and mentally. I had two pervasive feelings during my recovery from CFS: my legs often felt boneless and it was as if my mind were trying to peer out through fog. But once I set off, I knew there could be no turning back. I had to make it. I also had to put complete trust in an octogenarian to see me safely to the other side.

There were many of us on the walk. We set off at quite a pace behind Cedric, and then he stopped. In a very quiet voice he explained we must never get ahead of him, never go beyond the two assistants who were flanking him. Two blasts on his whistle and we must stop. That was it – he hardly spoke again for the next four hours. If anyone got out of line, he peeped his whistle and pointed, and the miscreant fell back to the group. It reminded me of the sheepdog competitions in the TV show *One Man and His Dog*.

After two or three miles we no longer felt as if we were on land; we were definitely 'at sea'. At every step the sand moved beneath us, and a lingering step could sink you. Most people walked barefoot with shoes slung around their neck. It was a glorious late spring day. As we passed the halfway point, what I can only describe as a transcendent silence fell.

Cedric indicated with one hand and one peep that we were to stop. This eighty-year-old man, with the tide times written on the back of his hand in biro, wearing rolled-up jeans, legs bearing witness to a life lived walking in jeopardy, reminded me somehow of Moses, or even Jesus, as portrayed in an old black-and-white film. The vast light of the bay was cinematic in quality, Cedric was undoubtedly charismatic, and we walkers were his devoted followers. (I know, I know – the jeans somewhat spoil my analogy, but there we are!) We were about to cross the deep channel of the river. We needed to stay together, to not stray beyond the boundary marked by 'brobs' – large branches of laurel that had been pushed into the bank to indicate the 'safety zone'. We were told to walk in one line, like a human hemp rope, an advancing army, looking out for the people on either side of us. We walked as one at the midpoint of 120 square miles of intertidal mud flats. As we strode down into the river channel, we naturally fell in step, the air charged with the swish, swish of well over a hundred people wading through waist-deep water, thrusting limbs forward against the tide – feeling simultaneously potent, conquering the tide, and only too aware of the vastness of the bay. The sound of legs marching through fast-flowing water will remain with me for ever. It was hard to forget the advice of someone at the start that this was the only place on the walk to pee – through your shorts. In among the sublime, we still have bodily needs.

It took a while before people started to chat again. Most of us were in our own space, reflecting on the power of this place and what this experience meant to us. For me it was a Rubicon crossed, full of hope. It was the ultimate test. I had waded through so much metaphorical dirty water to get to this point. I had survived and now I hoped to thrive. I was quite overwhelmed by the beauty and power of this moment. It was impossible not to think of religious symbolism of my chapel past – of immersion, baptism, a new life beginning – the power of water to transform. It was a moment of change, a test of my strength and determination to get well.

There were wading birds everywhere taking this twice-daily opportunity to feed. The silence was pervasive, save for the cries of oystercatchers. As we hit the firmer ground of the salt marshes near Grange-over-Sands I began to flag. Entering the town, my legs no longer felt attached to my torso and I wondered if I wasn't as strong as I had hoped – but then I saw the array of bodies, men and women, slumped on kerbstones, almost literally in the gutter, trying to find enough power to get themselves back to their cars. Walking eight miles is nothing; walking it on wet and shifting sand needs stamina. I'd made it, I could walk again. I was jubilant. If you'll pardon the pun, this day really did represent a line in the sand for me. I started to feel like I had no longer *vanished* in some shadowy quagmire. I was becoming visible to myself.

It was symbolic that I celebrated this moment in this place that I knew so well. I revisited those feelings of being young and free and full of excitement for the journey ahead. As I stood overlooking the bay, I could see the route of the train I took from Lancaster to Ulverston every morning of my first post-graduate teaching practice in 1980. It was a sweet memory of a very challenging time, a memory made sweeter still as I recalled the little trolley that served me a rescuing brew from a proper teapot on each homeward train journey.

Slowly I learned to trust my gut. I made new friends and reconnected with old ones. If I fancied a course or an activity, I'd sign up for it. I also tried a few things that were giving me cold vibes just so I could understand why they were not for me – curious as to what I could learn about myself from those things too, learning to be comfortable with being uncomfortable. In my local bookshop I came to trust my 'feeling' that this was *the* book I needed to read next, despite the fact it was in the gardening, engineering or even children's section. I started to embrace this freewheeling; a sort of other-worldly existence where I could follow my interests wherever they took me. It was like being a child again, except I didn't need to be home for tea and could afford more than a penny chew.

With my newfound beginner's mind I tried to look at the world with fresh eyes and good humour. I felt I had finally come to the point where I could start from scratch. I had found corners of my brain that I didn't know existed. I could sense a field of possibility opening.

5

STARTING FROM SCRATCH

The disempowerment and humiliation of older women is one of the most long-standing and unchallenged effects of patriarchy. As a result, ageing women are often engaged in an indecorous struggle to deny their experience and to act as if we were still young.

Uma Dinsmore-Tuli, *Yoni Shakti: A Woman's Guide to Power and Freedom through Yoga and Tantra*

At this stage in my story, I hadn't yet got out of the blocks. The cloak of invisibility certainly hadn't been replaced by a robe of wisdom. Of course, I wasn't really starting from scratch, I had a whole lifetime of experience to draw upon, but it was new territory and there was no map. I was adventuring.

One of the things I was looking forward to was attending the Hay literary festival. I hadn't solo camped since I was a teenager and I didn't think I could manage the family tent on my own, so I set off to the local camping shop to get a cheap, one-woman pop-up tent and camp bed. The fishing section had camp beds that also doubled as armchairs – perfect, I thought. I arrived at the delicious-sounding Gypsy Castle Campsite, excited and pleased with myself. The tent was up just ahead of the rain coming in, but I discovered a fatal flaw in my decision-making when it transpired that the bed-chair was too long for the tent. I would need to sleep with the foot end hanging out in the field or abandon the camp bed and sleep on the ground. To complicate things further, I'd had root-canal dentistry the day before. What could possibly go wrong? At first all seemed well, but it was, of course, in the middle of that first night, with the rain pouring down on my half-in, half-out sleeping arrangement, that my tooth started to throb and the throb turned to torture. I only had one pain killer in my rucksack. My thoughts turned to the tool kit in the car. Were there any pliers in there, or a hammer? But I didn't want to wake up the sleeping campsite by slamming car doors. It seemed a very long way to the Portaloos, and it was too wet to sit outside and make a hot drink. That night was long, cold and gruelling. It certainly did not give me any indication that something auspicious was about to happen. I was first in the queue at the pharmacy the next day, had a telephone conversation with my dentist and then dosed myself up with pain relief for the rest of the week.

One of the talks I attended was given by the writer and naturalist Stephen Moss, speaking about his book *Wonderland*. He mentioned that he had recently taken over as course leader for an MA in Travel and Nature Writing at Bath Spa University, and a little fire was lit that I was drawn towards. I went up to get my book signed and asked him about the course. A few days later I had a follow-up chat via Skype. I didn't think I would meet the entry requirements; like most people I had written a lot for work, but I was almost a complete novice in terms of creative writing, whether fiction or non-fiction. I submitted some samples of my writing – I was embarrassed by what I had to offer, but my excitement at the thought of the course overrode any qualms. Next there was an interview, which I am certain demonstrated just how inexperienced I was, but I hoped that my enthusiasm would win the day. And perhaps I was right, as I was offered a place.

Starting that course in the autumn of 2017 took me straight back to the excitement I felt as an undergraduate, more than forty years before. I walked up the gravel drive into Corsham Court, home to Bath Spa University's creative arts courses, peacocks cawing all around, into the splendid Elizabethan manor house. The building was glorious and set the tone for this very special time in my life. The rest of the students arrived, and we all fidgeted with our new stationery. We introduced ourselves and I soon realised that all the others were much more experienced writers than me and some were published already. Mostly their academic studies were in the recent past and I hoped I would be able to hold my own.

Undeterred, I took a deep breath, reminding myself that I was here to have fun and learn. It was refreshing to be back in a mixed-age group, and they were such a great set of characters. The lectures on setting up websites, writing blogs and getting published all sounded so fanciful and unlikely that I decided to just enjoy the course. I just wanted to write and relish the ride.

My 'beginner's mind' mentality served me well. I embraced singing to the trees, writing sounds, tastes and colour. I went off on my bike armed with paint charts to help me describe the autumn fields and woods. I gleaned snippets of conversations heard in coffee shops and wove them into longer stories. I took lots of risks with my writing – I wanted to test myself in every way. I experimented with poetry, multimedia, imaginary interviews with the living and dead, cocktail recipes about the meaning of life, whatever entered my quirky brain as it appeared. I wrote about the trees in my local woods and my newly dug pond. Many of the motifs were about dragonflies, emergence and taking flight, reflecting my inner life.

I also started to write about the lives of women, some known to me and others who I heard about. About the lives of women and girls I met in South Africa in 2006 who were living with HIV and AIDS. About an international community of women who were knitting prosthetic breasts for their unknown sisters recovering from breast cancer. At the same time, my travels started to focus on journeying among women, deepening my understanding of their lives and mine.

Given my love of travel, it is perhaps not surprising that the 'room of one's own' celebrated by Virginia Woolf took the shape, in my case, of a second-hand VW T4 campervan – a home conversion that the previous owner had decided to call Mr Binks. Picking it up from a local garage, ready to get going, I excitedly filled it with diesel and then watched in dismay as the fuel gauge sank and fumes filled the van. Whoever had converted it had drilled through the top of the petrol tank! The previous owners must have only ever run it at half full. Even with a new tank fitted, every so often I would drive over a rut and the gauge would drop to empty. Sometimes it would shoot up again when I hit another bump and I would be left guessing how much fuel I had. This was not reassuring – especially in the wilds of Scotland, for example. Mr Binks was endlessly breaking down and cost me more than its value in repairs. Eventually I sold it. I can only hope the new owners have reaped the benefit of all I spent on it. I bought a newer model and, touch wood, have had no problems. With my van and a folding bike, I can go anywhere.

It was during this period that I decided to take care of my mental health with psychotherapy. It's the hardest work I've ever done – seeing oneself emotionally naked, stripped bare of the constructs and projections we use as defences, can at times feel epic. Like a long climb up a mountain, it is not for the faint-hearted, but there comes a point when the path starts to undulate, when you reach the view that rewards you with perspective and hope.

I also wanted to improve my core physical strength, but after several amusing and embarrassing attempts at ballet, yoga and Pilates I still hadn't managed it. Then, during one very long drive home from northern Scotland, I got stuck on the M6 for what felt like several months of my life. My body crumpled and it took several physiotherapy sessions to straighten me out. The physio recommended that I try a different form of Pilates using something called a 'Reformer'.

As luck would have it there was a new Pilates studio in my small town. Walking through the door I was stunned – there in front of me was the Reformer, a large, framed contraption, hung with straps and moving parts that looked like a cross between a medieval torture device and *Fifty Shades*! The frame holds the body safely and in correct alignment while offering support, resistance and challenge – great for someone like me who has a poor sense of my own body (even knowing my right from my left is a challenge). It's not for everyone, but this machine has helped me enormously with my core strength and I now refer to it in my head as 'The Great Reformer'.

One of the assignments for my MA course was to organise a self-directed trip, write about it and try to get it published, or at least pitch it to a publication. We were learning how to get our work 'out there'. I had a long-cherished affection for the BBC's Shipping Forecast. As a small child I remember listening to it from my land-locked home on Salisbury Plain. I'm not sure if it was the signature music that drifted me off to other shores – how could it be? Ronald Binge's 'Sailing By' was only played at the midnight forecast, when I would have been long tucked up in bed, and yet it is there, stored in memories of my childhood, alongside my teddy and favourite apple tree. Perhaps it was the strictly prescribed, yet somehow unexpected, rhythm and cadence of the forecast itself. My family didn't travel far and so my knowledge of geography was hazy to say the least, but the sounds of 'Dogger', 'German Bight', 'Fair Isle', 'Faeroes', 'Hebrides', 'Viking' and 'Southeast Iceland' were captivating. Perhaps the enigmatic language – itself backing and veering like the wind – appealed to me. And weather events seemed to have echoes in my childhood life: *imminent*, which I heard as *immanent*, like God; *soon* (like lunch); *later* (like just about everything else); and even *poor becoming moderate* (aspirational, like my family).

As soon as the task was set, I knew where I wanted to go – off to the Faroe Islands. I had made solo business trips to far-flung places over the years, which didn't faze me at all, but my journey to the Faroes was different. This was my first proper solo trip, not coming under the 'work' or 'family' umbrella that had defined my travels for more than forty years.

The Faroe Islands sit halfway between Iceland and Norway, at 62° N in the North Atlantic. The archipelago is made up of an arrow-shaped arrangement of eighteen small islands, some connected by sub-sea tunnels or bridges, others only accessible by boat or helicopter. I spent the first few days as a tourist. I loved the capital, Tórshavn, with its welcoming cafés where I could sit, write and order my thoughts. I was intrigued by the ways in which the Faroese are embracing new approaches to sustainability – turning salmon skin, a by-product of the salmon fishing industry, into 'leather' for making shoes and bags, for example. Knitting shops and woollen wear was plentiful and I enjoyed the folk tales behind the unique patterns. I drove many miles from island to island, captivated by their unique culture and world view. Huge construction work was going on to create a sub-sea tunnel, including the world's only sub-sea roundabout, the 'Jelly Fish', linking the islands of Streymoy and Eysturoy.

I visited the Faroes in late April 2018, before the visitor season had started. There was a knitting festival, Bindifestivalur, in Fuglafjørður and I had arranged to interview the organisers in the hope that I might be able to use it for my assignment and to pitch to publications. The festival required huge amounts of organisation. Women had come from all over the North Atlantic, from Greenland, Denmark, Norway, Iceland, Shetland and North America. I was the only delegate from England, and one woman had travelled from Australia. There are no hotels in that part of the Faroes, so everyone stayed with local families. We had a choice of workshops, walks and entertainment – think Hay Festival with yarn instead of books! What I enjoyed most was meeting all these strong women, raised in fascinating and challenging climates. It was possible to piece together, in the style of psychogeography, how the skill and craft of knitting had travelled by sea across these remote land masses. Like yarn itself, the sea linked communities to their heritage, stitched together in garments of protection over hundreds of years. Conversations about the colours, patterns and stories that were knitted into garments gave me a greater understanding of the unique culture of the North Atlantic, where even today if a fisherman is lost at sea, he is often identified by the pattern on his gansey.

It was early on a Sunday morning when I drove from Fuglafjørður to Borðoy island via the seven-mile sub-sea tunnel. Mine was the only car in it. It was unnerving driving 490 feet below the sea, and at one point, when lights began to flash across the roof of the tunnel, I was scared silly – what did it mean, what was I being warned of? Should I stop? Claustrophobia gripped me and I just kept heading to the exit. It turns out the flashing lights were supposed to be a reassuring celebration that you were at the lowest, halfway point in the tunnel, and that now you were heading up and out! A roadside café as I reached land welcomed me with brunch and a place to compose myself.

I lingered a while writing, reflecting, and hoping the rain would stop. At 11am a live church service was piped into the building. Although I couldn't understand Faroese, the tone was very familiar – a melancholic pedal organ playing doleful hymns, a man's voice full of woe and thunder; but of course that might be projection on my part after a childhood spent in similar services. I asked the server about it. 'It's the only way we can stay open,' she said. 'No shops are allowed to open on the island on Sunday, just this café, but the religious service must be heard.' Many Faroese belong to, or are descended from, the Plymouth Brethren, Protestant followers of John Calvin, and their beliefs are still strictly adhered to on many islands. I returned to this café later, as indeed it was the only place open on the island all day.

I wrote my assignment on the flight home. Gail Simmons, the course lecturer in travel writing, encouraged me to enter it into *The Telegraph*'s 'Just Back' competition. Strangely, I had just boarded a flight to Corfu for a holiday with my wife when I received the email to say that mine was the winning entry for that week. The flight attendant told me to switch my phone off before I had chance to double-check I hadn't imagined it! Nine months later I found out that my entry had been chosen as the overall winner for 2018. It was more than a little boost to my confidence and emerging sense of self. I include the piece (overleaf), exactly as it was printed on the *Telegraph* website, not to show off (oh, alright, maybe just a little bit – sorry) but to reflect on how these five hundred words summed up so precisely my psychological state at the time.

This was not a conscious piece of existential writing – I was writing to fulfil the criteria for the travel writing element of the course. Neither was I trying to lay my soul bare to the world. I was writing about real fog but describing my inner fog. Who was I? Was my identity bound up with family and my gorgeous granddaughters? How was I defining myself now? Was I a writer, an adventurer or traveller? Or simply just having a nice holiday? Did I need to label it, or just enjoy it?

My solo trip to those other-worldly islands was, with hindsight, a turning point in my life. I did not know it then, but those islands would give me permission to unlearn. Unlearning is vastly undervalued – not celebrated at all, in fact. Learning is lauded, certificated, applauded publicly. So many of us keep and hold close what we 'know'. But it often turns out that what we *know* is in fact an opinion, or simply incorrect. Even science, so often lauded as 'things known', is a process of unlearning, finding out the new, replacing the old – and, quite often it turns out, 'proving' what was known by our forebears in the 'pre-scientific' age. Human beings also have the capacity to hold on to what is 'known', for years, sometimes centuries, after it has been disproven or is no longer relevant to society. Think flat earth, the sun going around the earth, the subordination of women and people of colour. Humans can remain stubbornly resistant to unlearning long after the misguided belief still serves them.

The fog in my piece was not a writer's conceit or a motif, it was a real presence. I was alone, trying to find my way around in dense fog, setting off on hikes only to realise that it was impossible to know

Why the Faroe Islands needs 37 words for fog

w telegraph.co.uk • 11 February 2019 • 3:15pm

Amid a strong field, Jan Courtney has been judged to have written the best Just Back of 2018 in our travel writing competition. Here we republish her account of discovering the magical fog of the Faroe Islands, first published in May. She wins £1,000 in the currency of her choice from the Post Office.

'What are you doing here?' asked the man I stopped to ask for directions in Tórshavn.

Not the angry, 'What the hell are you doing here?' nor the inquisitive, 'I'd like to know more about your plans', but the 'Why on earth are you here now?'

'It's not summer,' he said.

That much I'd realised. Fog meant ours was the last plane to land that day, fly as they must up a fjord, wingtips close to the towering slabs of granite on either side. There are 37 words for fog in Faroese, and I'd landed in mjørkakógv (very thick fog), giving me an often frightening drive between the airport on Vágar Island and the capital city on Streymoy Island. Even the sub-sea tunnel felt mjørkatám (hazy).

Two days later the pollamjørki (sea-mist) had lifted and I drove the same route in glorious sunshine, this time my breath taken not by fear of driving over the edge, but by the view; as my granddaughter would say, it was 'massive'. For once she'd be right, everything was massive; huge fjords and vast mountains rising straight out of the fishing-boat-blue North Atlantic, peaks still covered in where the edge of the cliff was. I was travelling between islands surrounded by so many types of fog, most of which I couldn't name, let alone pronounce. It was help from other women that helped me find my way through. At the first lunch of the knitting festival I was befriended by Katrin and her sisters, who grew up on the Faroes

snow, outfields turning from drab to emerald as I drove. I could easily believe in the existence of the 'huldufólk', the elvish people who live in the sorrel-green stones.

Tórshavn, from the Viking 'Thor's Haven', is one of the smallest capital cities in the world. It's a delight to potter around; noteworthy shops, restaurants and colourful houses with medieval grass roofs, and importantly, Tinganes, 'The Thing', seat of the Faroese parliament since the Viking era.

I'd come in part for the Bindifestivalur, or Knitting Festival, in Fuglafjørður. If that conjures up a Miss Marple-like congregation, you'd be wrong. More than 200 gutsy women from across the North Atlantic including Iceland, Greenland and Denmark, were celebrating, sharing and preserving the history of the craft that had kept generations warm and loved.

With no hotels in Fuglafjørður, delegates were accommodated in private homes. Every Faroese home I visited, however modest, had a table to seat at least 12, because as my host said, 'We're not used to coffee shops and restaurants, we need room to enjoy eating and drinking with our friends and neighbours'. This is a small nation, self-sufficient and yet not isolationist, harnessing technology yet embracing the values that make its culture so appealing.

Heading homewards, the plane took off through the hjallamjørki (belt of fog) and I was struck by how my trip was a metaphor for travel and life; we move between fog, some mjørki (summer mist), some flóki (bank of fog) and illumination, seeing the beauty beyond and adjusting our lens as we do.

Reproduced with kind permission from The Telegraph

but now lived in Elsinore, Denmark. They invited me to join them for meals, at evening entertainments and on the organised hiking trips. Katrin was extraordinarily kind, meeting me after the festival in Gjógv, telling me about Faroese culture and taking me to remote places that would have been tricky to find on my own.

This began one of the greatest joys of travelling as an older woman: experiencing how welcoming, inclusive and open-hearted women and women's groups can be to other women on the road. We need to unlearn the notion that women are 'bitchy, tribal and excluding'. That is not what I or my fellow Juicy Crones are experiencing, whether travelling or staying at home. We champion each other, celebrate together, check in with each other during tough times and take inspiration from one another. Many of us are finding our way and enjoy sharing our new experiences – from the mundane, such as which is the best sleeping bag for bigger bums, to the profound, supporting each other through bereavement and loss.

When I chose to travel to the Faroes, I could not have chosen a location that more accurately reflected my inner turmoil. Where was my focus now? Was it my grandchildren, crafting, travel, writing or meeting new people? Did I need a focus at all, or was retirement about 'doing a bit of what you fancy'? This uncertainty was of course the point of my journey at that point – I was lost and alone (but not lonely). I needed to experience the veil of fog, the intense effort to see through to what lies beyond. In my new and unmapped country, it would have been sensible to find my way slowly and with self-compassion. I didn't, of course, I went hell-for-leather seeking understanding, reading every book I could lay my hands on, listening to other women talking, making connections, and then heading out to this wild and unforgiving place. It's funny, though, how others see our struggle. Occasionally someone will say of that Faroes article, 'Didn't you write that piece about knitting?' And I suppose the answer is that yes, I did. I am knitting my life, dropped stitches and all, to the cast-off row.

After I returned from the Faroes, gradually I found, metaphorically speaking, the things that fitted me. I gave all my suits to charity and replaced them, again from charity shops, with 'playing' clothes. My criteria were simply A: is it comfortable and B: does it make me smile? Anything else was now irrelevant. Meanwhile the writing course continued to be intense, challenging and wonderful in every way. I was especially grateful for the people I met there. We travelled together in every sense of the word, walking and writing in Sella in the Costa Blanca mountains and closer to home in the west of England. I made friends for life who I meet regularly for walks and talks in the hills, with lots of coffee stops.

I learned much on that course, and throughout this long journey. And one of the most important things I learned is that it is we who need to act. The sun does not rise – the earth turns. If we want to own this phase of our life, we need to be the generators of change. There are so many reasons why it best serves the world if we maintain the status quo. By changing, by being the earth revolving around our own sun (whatever that sun means to us), we are eclipsing other stars and causing cosmic ripples. We will disappoint our loved ones if we aren't available for baby-sitting or caring on demand, and shock them if we say no to cooking dinner; we will be seen as selfish for spending time studying for a degree or learning a new skill. The gossips will whisper 'she's a bit odd', because we dye our hair purple or start batting for the other side by taking a female lover. They will be scandalised that we want to end a perfectly good forty-year marriage. They will titter and sneer at the younger lover. We may well find ourselves saying 'yes' or 'no' to things that are in opposition to our nearest and dearests' needs for the first time in our lives.

So, brace yourself, haul out your shield of Athena and sally forth. It's much better for you and the people you love in the long run than antidepressants or gin.

It turns out there was a stranger within me – perhaps not a stranger, but a long-lost friend, someone I knew a long time ago but hadn't met for quite a while. She was sending me messages from the heart. That part of me that had for many reasons – some practical, some emotional – not come out to play for a long time. She had been there all along, though; her creative energy, spirit and quirky world view had not been lost but exiled. And my long-lost friend was most certainly 'free for the strangest adventures'.

6

HEARING VOICES

Finding other women like myself helps me to understand my place in the great pantheon of human experience, and I am always grateful to anyone who points me in the direction of a woman whose story I did not know.

Sandi Toksvig, *Toksvig's Almanac*

All the women featured in this book – in fact almost all the women I have ever known – have throughout their life demonstrated tenacity, leadership, loyalty, resilience, a cooperative work ethic, common sense, and ability in their chosen field. It is obvious that what stood between them and enjoying post-menopausal adventures was not their personal qualities, nor necessarily a lack of knowledge (although a demonstration of what to pack in a rucksack is always handy). It was something less definable, something deeper.

In her uplifting book *Three Stripes South*, Bex Band sums this up: 'It's a sad fact that I felt like I needed permission to do something that I'd always wanted to do.' Bex is a young woman who grew up in an era of much greater equality than my generation, and she has experienced fewer years of 'lamination'. I hope she has experienced less misogyny, though I'm not confident on that score. If *she* struggled to follow her dreams, then how was this crone to do it?

Initially *Juicy Crones* wasn't a project at all – I just found myself chatting to post-menopausal women I met in a serendipitous way, soaking up their wisdom, while I was out hiking in the hills, or camping, or simply sitting in a local café. Gradually I realised that I needed to meet more women and hear different voices, voices telling me how they had found their 'juice', what they were doing and how had they given themselves their own 'permission slip'. How would I find my tribe? I needed women I could relate to, women who inspired me, gave me permission to be me, even.

I'd had a little success with my writing, but more importantly I was starting to believe that I still had something to contribute. As my health improved and I got fitter, I continued with my adventures and frequently headed into the hills, sleeping in my van. Meeting other women my age, I enjoyed some of the most honest, frank and raunchy conversations I'd ever had. These were no-nonsense, don't give a damn, this is how it is conversations; it may not be comfortable, we told each other, but I'm not going to sanitise my truth anymore. Life is too short to pretend. It is truly refreshing and wonderful to be in that place. Now when I walk with my contemporaries, I love that we rarely spend time on small talk. We don't have time to waste – we go straight to the big themes of life.

Initially this was a personal quest. I wanted to meet up with women who were embracing their 'third act' with gusto. As I talked to friends, and then friends of friends, I began to identify common themes that I hadn't heard talked about before. I welcomed the wisdom of these women, but what became clear is that many of them, like me, had made the journey alone and felt they were 'odd' in their struggle. It felt to me that it was time to listen carefully to what they were saying and to get their voices heard, for the benefit of everyone who found themselves with this inner conflict.

I was reading extensively during this time, and although I appreciated the books on menopause and self-help titles, I found little that resonated with me about post-menopausal life. Having got through the long years of the menopause, then what? It's a cliché, but there is some truth in the adage 'you've got to see it to be it'. In my quest for positive role models I was looking for women, like me, who had either reached retirement or, through personal crisis, had given up their careers. Or women who felt that life had never offered them the chance to follow their dreams at all. Who could I learn from? How had they managed to transition into post-menopausal life – their 'second spring' – not just surviving but thriving?

An idea started to take shape in my head – a book that would celebrate women who had made the tricky journey through menopause, not seeing that as the end, but rather the beginning of their transformation into a new life. It was around this time that I read *Goddesses in Older Women* by Jean Shinoda Bolen, a Jungian analyst and Professor of Psychiatry who has written extensively about the inner life of the older woman. In it, she writes movingly about the depths of new energy, insight and wisdom that are waiting for women in their 'third act'. Jean describes the archetype goddesses found throughout history – 'the goddesses of transformative wrath, the goddesses of mirth and bawdy humor, and the goddesses of compassion. When you can tap into the energies of all three, and also have wisdom, you are an internally free woman and a juicy crone.' Thumbing a nose at the received perception of crones as desiccated hags – and with a nod back to the long-gone days when cronehood was associated with wisdom – the phrase 'juicy crone' made me laugh out loud. It really struck a chord with me and galvanised me in my search to find my tribe.

I emailed Jean to ask her permission to use the phrase in my nascent project. This was her reply:

> Hi Jay
>
> 'Juicy Crone' was a subtitle I came up with to counteract the usual adjective that preceded Crones, such as 'dried up and old'. I didn't trademark it or do any such thing and wouldn't have – what you are doing with it warms my heart. I did want the word 'Crone' to become an expression of honor and respect once again.
>
> Please take the name and run with it!
>
> With love, hope, perseverance, trust and gratitude!
> Jean Bolen

Jean had given me an extraordinary gift and I decided to do exactly as she suggested. I would take the name 'Juicy Crone' and run with it.

I set about putting the project on a sound footing. It was important that women could share their stories in a way that felt safe and over which they felt they had control. Of course, I wanted to produce an interesting and thought-provoking book, but not at the expense of the volunteers. Many women felt they had been exploited during their life, so the last thing I wanted was to add to that burden. I committed to paper my promise that their stories would be heard in confidence until they were ready to share them with the world – or indeed chose not to, as some did. I explained to each woman I spoke to that this would be an iterative process, with drafts going between us until they felt their voice had been represented accurately. None of us gets to post-menopause without having lived a lot of life. We all have events that shape and form us, many of which, however interesting, we may not wish to put in the public domain.

Once my terms and conditions were in place, I set about planning my own adventures: to travel, to write and to talk with women who wanted to make their voices heard. My plan was to go from north to south, starting in Iceland and heading down through northern Scotland, gradually south through mainland Europe and eventually ending in New Zealand. Some trips would be solo, others with my wife. I wasn't sure how long all of this would take, and there would be time at home with family too. There was no rush – this was my big adventure.

This was 2019. We saw in the new year with my brother and his wife in France, and I welcomed 2020 as a year that promised perfect, balanced vision! HA! I was *so* wrong! The start of the Covid-19 pandemic changed my quest altogether. Like many people in the UK, I spent the first lockdown enjoying a beautiful spring in the garden, waiting for the storm to pass. It was my elder daughter's words, 'Mum, it'll take two years before things start to get back to normal', that made me rethink my plans. If travel was to be curtailed for two years, I needed to find a different way to continue with the project. So, when restrictions allowed, I met up with women who lived within driving distance. Often this took the form of sitting two metres apart in a field.

As luck would have it, around this time BBC Radio 4's *Woman's Hour* invited contributions for 'Listener Week', in which all the topics covered were offered or requested by listeners. As it happened, Jenni Murray was about to retire and I was invited to talk to her about my experience of ending work and the *Juicy Crones* project. It was a light-hearted conversation that I enjoyed enormously. After that interview, many women got in touch to tell me how my experience of feeling lost and 'washed up' upon retirement resonated with them. They told me that 'Juicy Crones' felt like their tribe. This encouraged me greatly to keep going in my quest. BBC Radio London then contacted me to be interviewed by Jo Good on the afternoon show. Jo was really enthusiastic about the project and invited me to return when the book was written. I was spurred on by knowing that other women would be helped by hearing each other's stories.

The irony of writing a book about journeying and having adventures while living with the most severe restrictions on our movements since the Middle Ages did not escape me. Sometimes I accepted it with a wry smile, other times frustration got the better of me. In a burst of optimism I contacted Bradt to see if they might be interested in the concept, and was delighted when they responded to say they were. From a shout-out, 'Calling all Crones', in their e-zine, I received responses from across the globe. Fortunately for me, by then the world was used to connecting via video call and I managed to follow up on everyone who contacted me.

Most of the women had never met me before so it was important to establish rapport and trust. It's a big ask of anyone to tell their story to the world – I promised that they could withdraw at any point until the manuscript was submitted. It was a risky ride on my part, too. My intention was to retell these stories as authentically as I could. I tried to keep quiet during our meetings, letting the women speak with as little prompting or direction as possible. They were all encouraged to talk, with a few open-ended questions from me. I was born to a deaf mother, so I learned to listen for two. I spent my professional life listening to young voices, so listening to my own generation felt like a natural progression.

These are their stories – they have chosen what has made it on to the pages of their chapter and what has not – and I have turned their spoken words into manageable chapters, as close to their authentic voice as possible. Inevitably, in the telling, we revise and reflect on our stories and our philosophy on life. And as draft copies passed between us, women often said, 'I've been thinking about that, and I feel differently now – I now believe…' There has been a lot of soul searching, but a lot of laughter and fun too. In the way of things we were all changed in the telling.

Each of these women talked about the ways in which they gave themselves permission to do the things they wanted to do. One told me that she regularly stops and asks herself, 'Is this how I want to spend the time that I have left?' What is it we want to do with our precious time?

Every woman in this book has had to face a life-altering, irrevocable event. Without exception they have spent time and energy, and found self-compassion, in the face of these events to find a peaceful place within, allowing them to own a unique path into a meaningful cronehood. They have faced the things we all dread the most: receiving a life-limiting diagnosis, the death of a loved one, betrayal, divorce, violence, a financial crisis. None of these events is invited: they are grindingly painful and often frightening. They can, however, have a very beautiful and unexpected silver lining of transformation, if we allow them to. In a recent TED talk, Jean Shinoda Bolen described crisis as 'liminal time' in which everything changes, and everything is thrown in the air. With time, the crisis can lead to a reappraisal, and sometimes that reappraisal enables us to reconnect with our dreams and our authentic self.

And that's what the women in this book are sharing with us – their transformative experiences. Each of the Juicy Crones explores what worked for them during this time of transition: not just in the *doing* but in the *being*.

When I reached out to ask women to tell me their stories, I was careful to take time – lots of time. We have all arrived at this place after fifty years or more and it is not possible to summarise – or honour – that journey in a ten-minute interview. I have spent many hours with the women who have shared their stories here.

I gathered the stories in as gentle and organic a way as possible. Our conversations were recorded as we walked and talked or chatted over coffee or lunch. With only three of the women did I have to entirely rely on Zoom interviews. Most women wanted to have their voice heard – but without exception they struggled with the tension between that and protecting their families. I was entirely guided by their wishes. Although, in every case but one, it was I who wrote the stories, I wrote them in the first person for immediacy and authenticity, and the tales that are told here belong to the women entirely. Reading their stories as they were being written, the women were invited to amend, revise and reflect. It was important that they should recognise themselves and could say, 'Yes, this is me' – only then was it signed off.

I learned from months of listening to women what wonderful storytellers they are – for them, so often story is not a linear process. Women tend to draw their history in; they gather and glean, and the telling of their stories is about understanding, about picking the ripest fruits, and about finding healing balms. Women's lives are cyclical; this is how we understand our world – lunar cycles, birth, death, rebirth. We have the potential to carry within us the next generation and hold it close. Getting in touch with this way of seeing the world is immensely rich, profoundly moving and deeply affecting. As each story unfurled, it was not uncommon for one or both of us to shed tears. The women shared stories of tragedy, violence and discrimination, but also of deep love, great excitement, wonderful friends and fabulous lovers. Of course, to protect loved ones, not all of it made it on to the page, but each story shines through with a deep, abiding honesty.

I hope that these twelve stories will encourage more women to speak their own truth, adding to the canon of women's voices. We need the canon to build and the cannon to keep firing. As Sandi Toksvig urges us in *Toksvig's Almanac*:

Capture the stories of the women in your life who may otherwise
go unnoticed in the passage of time.
Be active.
Write the wrongs of history.

History is created by those who write it down. I am proud that in some small way I have been able to contribute to women's voices being recorded.

These stories were not chosen because they were sensational, although many are. I was not looking specifically for women engaged in extreme ironing on Everest. We all love stories of derring-do, but rather than inspire, they can sometimes leave us with the feeling that the adventure being described is unattainable. We have the need for everyday heroines, those who have the audacity to lead their lives in the way of their choosing. What I found increasingly was that it is not the end or goal that is remarkable in any one story – it is the twists and turns of the path along the way. I was interested in women who had found their bliss or their flow despite – or perhaps because of – the obstacles they had had to overcome in order to be themselves. It became an evident truth that being a Juicy Crone is not goal orientated or a destination. The truths uncovered in these stories are more profound. They go beyond the 'judging' or 'measuring' part of the brain, leading us into metaphysics and the wisdom years that historically crones were respected for.

At least two of the women who contacted me had such remarkable stories to tell that they have since written their own books. Sandra Reekie was diagnosed with cancer in her mid-fifties and the prognosis was not good. Aged fifty-seven she decided, nonetheless, to follow her dreams, setting out on an intrepid solo journey to India. Her inspiring book *From YOLO to Solo* recounts her next journey of a lifetime, travelling through eight countries along the Silk Road and joining the pantheon of women who are making their voices heard through intrepid travel. Likewise, Joanna Moseley's remarkable feats on her stand-up paddle board, including paddling 162 miles coast to coast from Liverpool to Goole, led her to write *Stand-Up Paddle Boarding in Great Britain*. I love her self-descriptor – 'I'm a joy encourager, beach cleaner and midlife adventurer'.

Almost every woman who got in touch said in different ways, 'I wonder if you would be interested in my story… *but* it is probably not good enough – interesting enough – remarkable enough – to be included in the book?' This is something I do, too – apologise for myself, negate or minimise myself before I have even been heard –

and which I am trying to stop. I wonder why so many women do that? Are we still trying to make ourselves neat and small, to adopt false modesty, or take up less space in the world? Perhaps we judge our own stories –and therein madness lies – by a set of criteria that don't, when we examine them, resonate with us at all? We are, after all, the keepers of the stories we want and need to hear. The ones that resonate with the lives we have experienced.

These women were in the business of change, and as they told their stories they challenged their own thinking – and mine – constantly. They did feed back to me, however, what being involved in the project meant to them. They told me how they appreciated being listened to, that having their stories heard and validated allowed them to speak with honesty and integrity. Some reflected on how emotional and cathartic the process was, and how it instilled a sense of pride in what they had achieved. At the same time, they all expressed surprise to be included, and felt flattered – we all suffered from imposter syndrome. They all said in different ways that they didn't think that their story was worthy of a place in the book, but that everyone else's was exciting, inspiring and joyous! For many, telling the story was often the easiest part – reading it back was more challenging, and a few women at this point spoke of feeling very protective of loved ones. However, seeing their story written down reminded them of their courage to push through barriers, or not see them at all.

Of course, the stories of the twelve women in this book are a snapshot of their life when we met. Life may be very different for them now – we all change, we all evolve and grow. But here we have twelve expert witnesses. Whatever they are doing now, they are living the life of a Juicy Crone – this is their power. They are the voice of authority on their own life. Their inspirational stories offer us joy, hope and challenge and, most of all, capture the fun to be had in being a Juicy Crone. I hope that, like me, you will learn from them, and be inspired and enriched by them.

7

ALEX'S STORY:
POO(H) STICKS AT SIXTY

Perhaps what one wants to say is formed in childhood, and the rest of one's life is spent trying to say it.

Barbara Hepworth

As Alex unveiled her story, I got a strong sense of a her as a wild child growing up on a Somerset dairy farm, learning to speak fluent cow and running through the countryside with few constraints. Alex is not separate from nature but part of it – it is in her very being.

In April 2021 the Covid-19 lockdown had been partially lifted and I was able to meet up with Alex in Dorset for a walk. I set off in my van in snowy conditions on the day that campsites were allowed to open (although not their facilities – it was probably a good thing that the two-metre rule was in effect!). Alex had planned a circular route, and walking in the outstanding beauty of the downs above Bere Regis felt like the epitome of freedom for us both that day. These downs – an ancient landscape formed of chalk and clay and early agrarian endeavours – have been occupied since Neolithic times. Given its regal-sounding connections, Bere Regis was much smaller than I had expected. Thomas Hardy referred to it in *Tess of the D'Urbervilles* (lightly disguised as 'Kingsbere') as 'a little one-eyed, blinking sort o' place', but the countryside we walked through was anything but.

It was a glorious morning – sunny, crisp and clear. A coat-on, coat-off kind of day when you knew that spring had arrived. The sunken lanes, trodden since ancient times, were underlit with celandines and the woods were fringed with bluebells. Chiffchaffs were busy chiffchaffing and great tits were swinging on a nearby rusty gate. The irony did not escape me that later that week Alex would be running twenty-six miles in the Dorset Ooser Marathon, covering our path in less than half the time we walked together.

When Alex first contacted me to tell me of her Juicy Crone life as a trail runner, I couldn't help but see her in my mind's eye as a runner who was simultaneously hurdling over everything that life had thrown at her. She was excited about setting herself new challenges, including the possibility of running a solo ultramarathon. She was also facing a battery of medical tests. It would be far too easy to think of her as running to run away, to leave her painful and difficult situation far behind her. But as we ambled and chatted, it became evident that the opposite is true. Alex is running *to* life, as she graciously and thoughtfully revealed.

Nearing the end of our walk we headed downhill through the farmland of Black Hill and the wonderfully named Shitterton. As Alex's story tells us, life may sometimes take us to shittertown, but dark, muddy places are often rich in nutrition and offer us a place to develop roots and to grow in inspirational ways.

Since this piece was written, Alex was given the all clear in May 2022 and ran two ultramarathons for charity in the space of two weeks.

It all began when I was in my late fifties and my mother had a disabling stroke. While I was trying to care for her and sort out her estate I developed reactive depression. I'm always reluctant to take pills, so I decided to try a local parkrun to hopefully give me a lift. I'm not much of a joiner so it took quite a lot of courage, but I'm really glad I did. While I was looking after my mother and working as a teacher, running and looking after myself became more and more important to my health.

Around the time of my sixtieth birthday I joined an online women's group. I wanted to learn to embrace my whole female self. I wanted to feel more comfortable in my own skin, to be publicly myself, to no longer hide behind my masks. I'm a visual person and decided to explore the notion of masks graphically. My wife helped me to pour a bright blue latex mould over my face (with a breathing hole, of course). I've got photographic evidence! The whole experience was wonderfully revealing; I couldn't breathe properly, I felt panicky and trapped. I felt removed from the world; *I* couldn't be seen like that, and I didn't recognise myself. I realised that in staying behind the mask I was damaging *me*. I wanted to make friends with myself and learn how to be me. I didn't know at that point that just a few months later I would be facing a massive bombshell. In the peeling off I've discovered a core of strength that I'd previously stifled.

One of the things that happens on your sixtieth birthday is that the NHS sends you a neat little kit for do-it-yourself bowel cancer screening. You put a little piece of poo on a stick and send it to a laboratory for analysis. I completed the test but didn't think too much about it. I'd suffered a few digestive problems for a year or so but I hadn't thought them significant enough to worry about and, anyway, life was hectic, and I was recovering from Lyme disease. It was one of those things that you could easily put down to stress.

The poo stick test picked up some abnormalities and I was asked to attend a colonoscopy appointment. It was May 2017. I was alone when the oncologist delivered the devastating news that they had discovered a tumour and I had stage three bowel cancer. It was a moment of suspended reality. It hadn't occurred to me that I might need someone there by my side. My wife rushed in to be with me. She has been so supportive throughout the whole journey. We hadn't realised just what impact the news and subsequent medical procedures would have on both our lives – it's not just the person with the diagnosis who is affected. She has been my rock. The shock was horrendous. It was all too much for us to take in. I was completely numb and everything felt wildly out of control. I had a strong sense that the train had left the station and I was not the driver any more. Just two days previously I'd run six miles in a team event. It was hard to marry in my head apparently being so fit and well and yet having just been given this body blow of a diagnosis.

I was not prepared at all for that day. I never thought for one moment that it was cancer, and I will always regret not acting sooner by responding to those early, niggling symptoms. Hindsight is such a wonderful thing.

If anything about getting cancer can be called lucky, I was lucky that Sunseeker, a yacht-building company, had donated a robotic operating theatre to Poole Hospital and, more importantly, that I had a surgeon skilled in robotic surgery to operate on me. They removed about a foot of lower intestine, which took me some time to recover physically from. I was discharged in June 2017. Two months later I started a course of chemotherapy but unfortunately had a severe allergic reaction to it, and the oncologist advised me to stop the treatment because it posed a greater risk to my life than the cancer itself.

Once again I was in shock, but I knew I needed to face the huge existential questions that were in front of me. I needed to learn how to look after myself both physically and mentally or, as I feel it now, spiritually. This was my marker point, my moment of transition and transformation in many ways. It's a bit of a cliché, but this was the start of an awakening of *me*. The diagnosis, surgery and failed chemotherapy were devastating. My situation was horrible and frightening, and the awareness of it is always lurking in the back of my mind. Not being able to complete the chemotherapy course has left me feeling vulnerable, but I've learned to accept that it could have killed me. The chemotherapy made me more ill than my first surgery and the two major surgeries I later needed.

Wonderful though the NHS is, at that point in my recovery conventional medicine had nothing else to offer me and I began to research alternative forms of help close to home. What I'm about to say is not me offering medical advice – I'm not qualified to do that. But once the cancer specialists recommend I stop the chemotherapy, and in the face of no conventional medicine being available, this is what has helped me to live as healthily as I can and stave off the spread of the disease for as long as possible. Alongside my routine check-ups and advice from my doctors and cancer specialists, I have regular appointments with a nutritional immunologist and a medical herbalist. It helps me feel that I have a degree of agency. The regimen I try to follow is the keto diet, which is high in good fats, medium in protein, and low in carbohydrate. I've invested so much time, money and energy on this that it's been like studying for a PhD in my own personal health, fitness and well-being. It's taken me a couple of years to find the best balance of nutrition to support my body and lifestyle.

In addition to looking after my nutrition, I have found that running has had a profound effect on my well-being. It started the process of me reconnecting with myself. Running is a whole body and mind experience. Heart and gut. I find peace when I'm running. For me it's soul-enhancing – it makes me feel so alive. It's hard to explain, but I immediately connect with the 'little me', the one who ran wild around the farm, the one who was so happy, before we were forced to leave the land and everything was wrenched from me. Running allows me to be in a different realm, one where I feel part of the natural world, not separate from it. That in turns feeds my passion for the nature photography I enjoy while I'm out on my runs.

My first outings with parkrun were in my late fifties, but I really got the running bug after my cancer diagnosis and treatment. Strange as it sounds, it has been my antidote, my counterbalance to all the medical treatments and procedures, and became a big part of my recovery and my life change. I took on my first ten-mile race in November 2017, six months after the first surgery to remove part of my bowel. In April 2018, I ran my first half-marathon and optimistically signed up for an ultramarathon that summer – a total of just over sixty miles in two days. I paid for a few coaching sessions, which gave me a helpful training structure. I was loving learning to run. I joined my local running club in Dorset. I've made so many friends at the club, and they've been a huge support to me. Learning to look after myself during a race has been very important: I have to plan carefully, giving myself enough fuel without upsetting my digestion.

It was when I tried trail running that I truly reconnected with a deep love within. I always knew I was a trail girl, from my childhood trots around the farm – road running would never really be my thing. I find marathons too pressured, too competitive and (this will sound perverse) too *short*. It's counter-intuitive, I know, but ultramarathon trails seem more leisurely. The hours and miles stretch ahead and I don't feel any pressure to perform. I can take time during the sixty-odd miles to get into my stride and find my flow. There comes a sweet point in each event when I'm in my zone. And then the magic happens.

What I experience through trail running is difficult to put into words. I feel a magnetic draw, an uplift, a scent on the wind, and gradually as the miles go by I feel an unveiling. I glimpse possibilities and understandings. I feel a compulsion, I'm drawn to it, I have purpose – yet it's playful. I feel free and yet connected to the natural world. I'm no longer separate and there are no boundaries. I feel alive and completely myself. The traumas that I've held in my body for so long are given balm and I feel well. There is a wholeness, a oneness, and a demasked acceptance of who I am. It's mystical, elusive, transcendent. I feel a pull – a calling, even. I'm not religious, but long-distance trail running is a spiritual experience for me.

The other thing about trail running is that it allows me to take photographs. Documenting nature through photography is as important to me as the running itself, which is why I enjoy running alone as well as with friends. Running and photography are symbiotic pleasures for me – it's about me running in nature and capturing the picture, the essence. I'm still nuts about cows, dogs and horses, so they're usually in the frame. If I'm faced with the choice of a great picture or a better race time, I always choose the picture!

Ultramarathons are social events, and when we overnight in a tent it's like being at a mini festival. It's a whole new side of myself that I'm starting to enjoy. I'm normally a very private person – quite an introvert, really. Although I have taught in schools for years and volunteered to contribute to this book, I find talking, joining things, and social situations quite difficult. I've had to learn to accept intrusion into my body and I'm challenging myself to share my thoughts and feelings with others. I just want to get on with life, with living and with running. My running friends have been so supportive and caring as my running career has continued despite all the health setbacks, but even they don't understand the mental and physical toll it takes for me to bounce back after every surgery and every worrying test result.

By the summer of 2018, when I did my first ultramarathon trail run, I was feeling strong and confident. I'd beaten this thing even without the advantage of chemotherapy. Then, in the autumn of the same year, a PET scan detected a lung metastasis. It was very hard to stay positive and it floored me emotionally. I had keyhole surgery in November to remove that mass, followed by months of recuperation. But five days after coming out of hospital I walked alongside my running mates for a mile in a night race through a dark forest, wearing a head torch and a chest drain!

It's so hard when you're forced to drop out of these events.

In January 2019 I started training again, building distance, terrain and stamina, practising running with a loaded pack, and rehearsing mentally. Twenty-nineteen was such a good year. I had no visible signs of disease. With the support of my running coach I ran my second ultramarathon, 'Race to the King' – fifty-three miles from Arundel to Winchester. It took seventeen long hours but I was elated.

Living well with cancer is like riding a roller-coaster set on an adverse camber. In May 2020 a liver metastasis was discovered. In the middle of the Covid lockdown my fear of hospitals escalated; getting all the necessary tests and surgery done during the pandemic was distressing, frightening and, oh, so lonely. They removed the mass from my liver and, once again, I was faced with two months of recovery and building back my physical and mental strength. It's an intense experience, requiring huge amounts of determination, as well as acceptance and humour.

My medical team has been amazed by my recovery and my surgeon has used me as a case study at international conferences. I've also been featured in women's running magazines. Perversely, despite the surgery to remove a section of my lung, I have a greater lung capacity, thanks to my running, than most people do. Strange, but true! The body's natural ability to heal is incredible, but it needs patience and that's not my strong suit. I have an urge to keep going, a sense of there being no time to lose, which doesn't help me rest, recover or relax – whatever that means.

Running has become an increasingly spiritual activity for me, and that has allowed me to access the deepest parts of myself. I'm normally tightly sprung, like a jack-in-the-box. I stress easily and I'm aware that my explosive emotional self is often close to the surface. So, unlikely as it sounds, I've started to meditate. At first it was something I thought I *should* do, but now I know it helps me so much that I find I *want* to do it. After all these years I still wake early, even though there are no longer cows to milk. I spend thirty minutes when I wake up listening to a meditation app called Calm. It gives me a serene and focused start to the day. Then I pull on my running gear and get out into the wild as soon as possible. Running towards the sunrise I feel energised and uplifted. Greeting the dawn is more than a metaphor for me.

I also like to give forward as much as I can. In the last couple of years my running mates and I have raised money for Maggie's centres – drop-in centres for people affected by cancer – and for Bowel Cancer UK.

I dread the routine testing every May and November, but, wonderfully, in 2021 the blood tests, colonoscopy and MRI were all clear each time. I was so excited to be given the all-clear in May but disappointed that all the races I'd trained for and looked forward to had been cancelled because of the pandemic. I don't know how long I have left – none of us does – but the relationship I have with time means that I'm eager to take part in as much as I can as soon as I can. Inspired by other women, I decided to seize the day, and in June 2021 I ran part of the Race to the Tower route by myself – my first solo ultramarathon – without any of the usual infrastructure in place. A race of that length burns thousands of calories and gallons of water. This is ultramarathon the hard way: no water stations, no first aid, no loos and no accommodation. It was exciting and scary in equal measure. I booked a camping pod in Broadway, in the Cotswolds, and took a taxi to where the official start would have been. Two friends each ran a few miles with me to spur me on and Jay popped up every now and then in her van to offer snacks and water. But essentially, I was alone on a very hot day, demolishing my demons, as I ran up and down those challenging Cotswold hills. Despite the struggle I had several miles of inhabiting my zone, centred and running free.

I would never have chosen this path, and it sounds such a cliché, but having cancer has been the making of me. I was sleepwalking through life and now I'm living every moment to the full. It's exciting for me not only to find my voice but to make it heard.

8

DEBS'S STORY:
TEA IN HUNGARY

Transformation is rarely easy. At times, you may long to retreat to a less vital and more domesticated version of yourself. But remember: the strength of the Earth resides within you, supporting you in your quest for wholeness.

Mary Reynolds Thompson, *Reclaiming the Wild Soul*

Debs was one of the women who responded to my shout-out in the Bradt e-zine of spring 2021. She wondered if I might be interested in her story of her new beginnings in Hungary. Like every other woman who contacted me, she doubted that her story was interesting enough to be told, and like the rest of us struggled with imposter syndrome as the story got closer to being printed.

Debs began to ask profound questions of herself as she journeyed through the menopause, starting what was to become a philosophical journey for both her and her husband, Mark. They have found answers in a unique and unexpected place. Setting up a business can be tricky; doing so in a country where you have to learn a new language takes bravery – and Brexit, a global pandemic and war in Europe have added many more layers of complexity to their adventures. Despite all of this, they have kept going, managing to make a welcome haven for guests while simultaneously finding meaning in what Debs describes as 'the autumn of our lives'. That phrase can have negative connotations, but Debs describes this time in her life as the season when everything has come to fruition. She has gained great insights and a rich, fulfilling – juicy, even – experience of menopausal life.

Life is long and through it we live several lives. It was important for me to realise that, to allow myself to be inspired to *have* other lives. I have always loved my work, but when my children left home I thought, surely this can't be it? I really feared that I would be left looking for things to fill the time. It took me a while to orientate myself. I still felt I had plenty of adventure in me, but I wasn't sure of the direction of travel. I think the whole process of menopause prompts women to ask huge questions. Who was I at this stage in my life? What did I *want* to do, rather than what *should* I do?

The cold fact was that I needed to continue to work in the UK until I got my pension. As an accountant I had advised and helped many people to realise their dream of setting up a small business. I had witnessed their hard work and risk-taking, but also the joy of creating something of their own. Having a vision of the future, making it happen through your own ingenuity and hard work, as they did, and enjoying the rewards appealed to me. My husband, Mark, and I realised that we wanted to give ourselves that same opportunity – to set something up for us. But were we brave enough?

We had long planned to travel when we retired in 2023, but as that time drew closer we started asking the 'then what?' question. What would we do when we returned from our travels? Would the same questions be waiting for us when we got back to the UK? It just felt too soon to be winding down.

Mark and I are completely different characters – he is very steady and I'm a bit of a grasshopper – but we both started to feel that travelling wasn't going to be enough for us. I could also see the possibility of some conflict arising: I would continually want to see the next place, but he would be happy to stay wherever we were. We had been working on converting a minibus into a motorhome for quite some time, so we were all ready for the off, but we both felt we wanted to do something else before we drove off into the sunset.

We were throwing ideas around between us and then one day a campsite appeared for sale on Facebook! The campsite was in Hungary, not somewhere we had ever thought of visiting, let alone somewhere we might set up a business. I just laughed about it and didn't give it a second thought. But, as he was driving his lorry the next day, Mark did. It was really exciting and inspiring him. When he got home, he asked if I had been thinking about it. I hadn't. We decided we would consider it and within five minutes I'd booked two flights to Budapest for £20 return on Wizz Air!

So, there we were in February 2020, boarding a plane for Hungary, with absolutely no idea of what to expect. We knew the location was in an unspoilt 'wild' region, but we'd need to research our journey.

Driving from Budapest airport to the campsite, we passed Lake Balaton – famous for watersports, the lake is vast, with far-reaching views disappearing into the horizon. About a thirty-minute drive further on we came to the Koppány Pines campsite, an oasis down a single-track road with its own hill to climb, and woods and rolling hills beyond, stretching for miles. On that first visit the air was thick with the humming of bees and other insects; Hungary is famed for its fabulous butterflies, but they were yet to be revealed to us. The meadows of the campsite and lakes in the distance lay below us. We did not yet know about the traditional vineyards and press houses and all the many small local producers that were later to become part of our life.

As we stood looking down across the valley, we turned to each other smiling – we both knew this could be a special place. With an amazing feeling of calm, we felt we had found a home. We looked at each other and said, 'Yeah, let's do it!'

Koppány Pines campsite is situated in the Koppányvölgy Natúrpark. It's about an hour and a half from Budapest, set in the superb, unspoilt Koppány Valley. The park's hiking trails run right past the site, there are cycle routes, and it is perfect for horseriding. There are also three thermal spas close by, ideal for relaxing at the end of a long day of walking and cycling. It was a landscape that spoke to us, and we hoped it would attract other nature lovers, too.

We knew we didn't want to get into debt for any venture; we felt that getting a loan, especially at our age, was just too risky. So many small businesses fail – around one in five every year in the UK. As it was too soon for me to retire, in order to reach our goals we accepted that we would need, for a while at least, to live separately. My partner funded the purchase of the campsite out of his savings and at first he would run it, aiming to turn a profit as soon as possible. Mine would have to be a slower transition: I still had commitments in the UK so I needed to remain UK-based, spending only the camping season in Hungary, until our plans came to fruition. We had a finite amount of money and we accepted from the outset that we were taking a risk. My father always told me never to gamble more than you can afford to lose. We were determined to succeed, but we were also grounded in reality. We might not be successful, we knew, in which case we would have to write the venture off as one *very* expensive holiday.

It is important to keep your feet on the ground and be pragmatic about the risks you are taking. This is always the case with being an entrepreneur but, logically speaking, the older you are, the less time you have to recoup losses. On the other hand, with age one does gain wisdom and pragmatism. We went into the project with our eyes open, but more importantly with a sense of adventure.

Very luckily for us, the owner of the local pub in Koppány is from Nottingham. We talked to him a lot before we committed to the campsite. We got on with him immediately and he has been so helpful in introducing us to the neighbours and helping us understand local customs. The locals have also been lovely. So helpful – even going so far as to bring tractors over to help us lift and shift stuff. Our neighbour opposite, well into retirement, came round most mornings with pálinka (the Hungarian hooch!), a traditional welcome in Hungary, and everyone has been trying to help us with the language.

My family of origin was nomadic. We moved all around the world for my parents' work, so living abroad is in my veins, but for my husband it is new territory and a big step. It would be a test of our relationship, too: how we each coped with living, working and creating a business at this stage of our lives, across two countries.

It has to be said that it was an unlikely choice: Hungary isn't a usual holiday destination for the Brits and we certainly knew very little about it. We couldn't read the road signs and we couldn't understand the language. Luckily, because of my upbringing, I am good at understanding the gist of foreign languages. We both set about learning Hungarian straight away. Mark has been focusing on the spoken language with Duolingo, and I have been concentrating on trying to understand the written word. My earliest attempts were with the local guys in the pub – before I realised that it was frowned upon for women to be in the pub! – where we had a conversation by passing my phone between us using Google Translate.

Hungarian is a very interesting language. It is neither Slavic nor Indo-European. It has its roots in a northern nomadic culture, probably structured in the first century BCE when tribes began to settle, and is part of the Finno-Ugric, Uralic group of languages. It is phonetic, which helps, but has forty-three letters in its alphabet, which doesn't!

We had factored in how Brexit would affect our venture, but one of the risks we didn't anticipate was a global pandemic, or the terrible war waged on the people of Ukraine. The sale had just been finalised when the world was hit with Covid-19. Part of the deal had been that the previous owners, who were also from the UK, would stay for a while and teach us how to run the campsite, which was due to open for the season just a few weeks later. They promised to help us through the labyrinth of legal paperwork to make the transfers and transitions. Unfortunately, because of the pandemic, they went straight back to the UK when lockdown was announced. And for us the pandemic meant we didn't actually get to the campsite until July, rather than May as we had planned.

Once we had taken the plunge, the challenge was to jump over the seemingly impossible number of hurdles that lay before us. Every task seemed knotted in bureaucracy which, as in every country, is couched in official language that was hard to understand. We started to feel overwhelmed – and then we took a breath, paused, and made ourselves reframe the situation. We needed to find balance; this was supposed to be our adventure. We needed to laugh at the things that went wrong, learn from our experiences and take pleasure in our victories, even if it was just sending the right form or saying the right thing to the right person! We agreed to enjoy each challenge, even if things went wrong.

Things do go wrong, things can fall apart, but every time this happens, I learn something new. We are learning so much about ourselves, but also the hospitality business, about life in Hungary and, most importantly, about ourselves as a couple and as individuals.

To enable me to join Mark for the camping season, I reduced my workload and took in lodgers. Never did we imagine that at our age we would be living with lodgers! We learned as much as we could from other people who had set out on alternative lifestyles. We devoured every TV programme we could from *Four in a Bed* to *A New Life in the Sun* to *Escape to the Chateau*. We are hungry to gain as much as we can from the experience of others, even if it has been dramatised for the small screen. And we are determined not to gloss over their challenges – we glean so much from their experiences. We can learn vicariously what problems might beset us and learn too from the inevitable relationship issues that crop up when you are trying so hard to make a new life. Television often doesn't show the tough side of things, nor when ventures fail altogether. However, we have been inspired and encouraged by these programmes.

When people book to stay with us, whether in the guesthouses, camping or in our 'nature reconnection' wild glamping tents, we hope they feel as if they are sharing a part of our life, our experience. We are not aiming to create a sanitised holiday 'resort'. This isn't just a campsite, it is our dream, and we love telling people about it, how we are making our dream a reality. Many people have a fantasy to do what we have done, so we try to be as honest as we can with them.

The campsite was quite run-down in the beginning, so we set about making it welcoming and comfortable. This is a beautiful, wild part of Hungary – we wanted Koppány Pines to reflect that, and for our guests to have the experience of being in nature but also to be comfortable while they drink in the wonder of this place. It's a rural community. The villagers live a humble country life that revolves around family, friends and simple pleasures. My abiding image of the place is of people in their gardens tending paprika plants. It's a peasant's way of life and quite outside our experience. The locals forage for food in the forests. It's not trendy and doesn't require designer wellies or waxed coats. It's just how it has always been done.

We completely renovated the guesthouses, using recycled, original furniture wherever possible. We have also renovated an on-site caravan, which we have situated on a ledge with amazing views. For those choosing an immersive wild experience, the bell tents offer the option of being in the meadow, overlooking the valley, where the deer roam freely.

As our love for this place has deepened, we have tried to make each guest space as close to nature as possible, but indulgent too – after all, our visitors are on holiday! They can order breakfast hampers to be delivered to their porch and we are around during the day to make sure we help to make this a very special time for them. We want them to take home wonderful memories of being in nature and a renewed sense of self.

Once we had got the fundamentals of the campsite and guesthouses operational, it dawned on me that I still didn't feel I had something of my own here. I really wanted to put my mark on the place, to unleash my creative energies to celebrate this new phase in my life.

When I was perimenopausal I developed horrendous symptoms: fungal infections, raging temperatures, foggy brain, intense itchy skin, exhaustion. I was reluctant to take prescription medication and certainly didn't want to take antidepressants, which is what I was offered. It was all quite frightening. One of the things that really helped me was experimenting with herbal teas. I am not a herbalist, but I know from experience that whatever symptoms I was experiencing, I could source a herbal tea that improved how I felt and enabled me to feel like *me* again. Hungary is famous for its thermal baths and our campsite is conveniently located near three of the best – Igal, Tamási and Dombóvár. The thermal Lake Héviz is also close by. This set me on a train of thought and inspired me to set up a wellness infusion tea house. I wondered if other guests, especially women, would benefit from herbal teas in the same way I have.

We trialled the tea house in season two and it has proved very popular. Women appear to be more open to the benefits, but interestingly also families enjoy the idea of collecting herbs and sharing family time with a pot of freshly steeped herbal infusion. I am really hoping that in time the tea house will provide a place for local women to meet, as well as for visitors to enjoy the healing properties of the herbs.

I was unable to resist bringing the very British institution of 'afternoon tea' to Hungary, so now we offer homemade jams and bakes with local botanicals to accompany the infusions and tisanes. Of course, I include scones and cream too. We also offer traditional Hungarian nights where we showcase Hungarian kettle-cooking with story-telling, stargazing and wine tasting. All our produce is either grown ourselves or brought in by local small suppliers. We like to include and support the local community as much as we can and welcome them alongside our campers.

The concept of botanical wellness fits perfectly with life in a nature park, and I aim to grow most of the herbs for the infusions. The herb garden is shaped like a leaf, which I hope will be picked up by the Tourism Bureau's drones that fly overhead – cheeky, I know! I have set to and created herb beds that look like real double beds, which make me smile every time I see them. I've never grown a thing in my life, so it has been a big learning curve. When my first aubergine grew, I felt like I had given birth to another child! I keep reminding myself that the small experiences are actually big, and part of my adventure.

We have experimented with many activities for our guests, including making wood-fired pizzas, treading grapes and stargazing with a telescope on the tea terraces – the skies here are unpolluted by lights, and it is quite magical. After many evenings missing our own mealtimes because guests wanted to sit and chat with us, we decided to turn it to our advantage and offer 'dine with the host' opportunities. People enjoy hearing about our experiences and reflecting on their own dreams.

I have come to understand that Koppány Pines is a healing place for me. I hope that we have been able to create opportunities for our guests to experience its restorative powers too. As I spent more time in the nature park – walking in the woods, being among animals and birds and spending so many hours outside – I realised that it was wonderfully good for my health. I sleep so well there. Walking in the woods, being among animals and birds and spending so many hours outside really improved my health. When I returned to the UK after the first season, I wanted to maintain that feeling and started forest bathing. Forest bathing is more than just a 'walk in the woods': the aim is to give the mind a chance to find an oasis of calm. Switching off all devices, breathing deeply and consciously directing thoughts away from day-to-day worries and routines, I focus on my senses as I walk, slowly taking in the smells, sights, sounds and tastes in the air. It isn't the same in the UK, where it is hard to escape road noise; initially, I found this background drone quite distracting. But mindfulness in nature is about using your senses and not prejudging your surroundings. It's about inviting your mind to immerse in whatever nature is around you. I love the calm this brings, and over the winter of 2021 I trained in nature connection mindfulness in the UK. I am now able to offer mindful photography and forest bathing to guests in Hungary. It's all part of the vision of this becoming a nature wellness centre and of sharing the peace that being here gives us. My path has also inspired Mark to pursue his interest in bushcraft and also train to teach.

One of the biggest challenges for me in this whole venture has been taking time just to enjoy the ride and to do the things I *want* to do. After all, we both decided to take the plunge as an active choice. I am trying very hard not to feel as if we have just moved 'work' to a different location. This was something for us to *enjoy* as well as work hard at. It's so important to remember that each moment in life is unique and must be savoured – it's too easy to rush past these significant times. I am reminding myself to embrace this part of my life, and the more I visit the more embedded I feel in a new way of being. My word for 2022 was 'reflection'. Not just to keep striving forward but to take time to reflect on the things I have done and achieved, and to enjoy the memories again and again.

As we get older, I think we are less fearful of change. We can more readily shed our skin and understand that it's time to move on, time to grow a new skin. But work habits are hard to change, and I am really trying to give myself permission to be 'selfish'. That is, to enjoy doing the things I want to do. Women are built to please, but I am learning that I need to have boundaries too. That's a huge shift in my sense of self: that I can own my life and make choices that suit me. Of course, Mark and I are there to serve our guests, but it is our dream too. Having said that, we have had many wonderful reviews from guests, and that is hugely rewarding. It sounds paradoxical but I have never felt so excited, nor so content, about my life.

This has been an enormous adventure for both of us. I have stepped far out of my comfort zone of accountancy and explored my creative side. For years I have longed to 'do my thing'. Never did I dream that 'my thing' would be setting up a wellness tea house and nature reconnection guiding in rural Hungary! But there you are – you never know what you can do until you say 'yes' to something that is calling you.

9

ANDIE'S STORY: 'LOWER THE NOSE'

The only way to get rid of the fear of doing something is to go out and do it.

Susan Jeffers, *Feel the Fear and Do It Anyway*

The car park of the Cotswold Water Park doesn't spring to mind as a place to think lofty thoughts about the excitement and romance of flying. The café and facilities are closed due to Covid restrictions, but here Andie and I are sitting on a patch of grass under a crab apple tree. I've taken two picnic chairs from the back of my van and opened the folding table, which ensures that we stay the regulation two metres apart. It's 2020, we've just come out of the first lockdown, and finally I can start meeting Juicy Crones in person. It isn't quite the 'journeying' across continents that I'd envisioned when I first dreamt up my Juicy Crones quest, but there's a deep joy in being away from the confines of home. I'm craving seeing friends and family again.

Andie has readily agreed to meet me halfway between our respective homes. I had intended to meet and talk with her at the flight school, and maybe even go for a fly with her, but the school is still closed. So I invite her to tell me the story of how and why she learned to fly. As she speaks, it occurs to me that Andie's experience of needing height or distance to gain perspective is a common theme for many Juicy Crones. There is clearly wisdom to be found in being up in the clouds or high on the hills.

I'm about three thousand feet above the ground, but my mind doesn't tarry with the vulnerability of the situation. I feel powerful up here and those feelings in turn empower me. I allow the sensations of flying to course through me, feel what it is to soar. I feel strong and focused. I feel as if this is what I was born to do – to fly a plane.

I'm in the zone. This is where I'm *me*. I have thirty-four hours of flying under my belt, which is a massive achievement for me. I'm confident and calm and have a sense of my whole being. But it's busy up here – you really have to concentrate and constantly be monitoring your instruments and what you're doing. I can now recognise how the engine should sound at a given stage of flight without referring to the airspeed indicator. It's good to feel in tune. When the instructor is silent, that's a good sign. I have control. It's thrilling, absolutely exhilarating!

I'm doing this for me. I'm not sharing myself with anyone else. It's not a relational experience – I'm no longer Mum or Grandma, a wife or a daughter. I'm out of reach while I'm up here. I can't be contacted. I'm alone with my thoughts and I try to keep it that way until well after we've landed. I love the speed, the view – I love the feeling of *I can do this*. It's a relationship with the aeroplane. It will fly for me if I let it.

Despite having passed technical exams on the physics of how aeroplanes fly, it still feels hard to believe that it can be possible. There is more than a little magic to it. Here I am in a small metal fuselage with two wings at right angles, a propellor driven by an engine and a set of wheels, simply using the laws of thrust and lift to get us airborne and flying away from the airbase. We're cruising at ninety-five knots. It's just me flying the plane. On a clear day the landscape stretches out all around and everything is in its place – not moving, just there. Time changes at that height – it has a different dimension, and the terrestrial hour transforms into celestial time. It's quite beguiling.

With a father in the RAF, I spent my childhood moving from one RAF station to another, never really feeling at home. I was eight years old in 1965 when I first went on an aeroplane, flying to Norway with my parents. What I remember are the physical sensations – the speed of the plane powering down the runway, the roar of the engines – it was thrilling. I remember the feeling of being pushed back into the seat, the thrust holding me there with its immense power, slightly winding me. It was in that moment that I thought, 'I want to fly when I grow up.' It was a dream that kept rising – and then getting pushed down. Even today those feelings come back to me when I'm flying.

It's quite difficult to accept that this dream, these feelings, this ambition, was there in me more than fifty years ago. I have to pause to take that in. I'm stunned by the realisation – wistful even. Regret is a tangled emotion.

It's hard to determine why my dream didn't come true and why I didn't set my mind on becoming a pilot. For one thing, I'm not sure I even shared my dream with my parents. Did I put words around it? Did they know this was what I wanted? Did I articulate this out loud? I'm not sure. I have a brother who is eight years older than me. He was very able and went to Cambridge to read law, then became a partner in a London law firm. I love him dearly but I think he cast an exceptionally long shadow over the young me. I didn't feel able to compete, or think I could be as successful. I'm not sure if these feelings were unique to me or developed within my family setting, or if it was a societal norm that boys, especially first-born sons, should be the high-flyers (if you'll pardon the pun).

My mother once said to me, 'You're a jack of all trades and master of none.' I was hurt by that. I think she just meant that I never stuck at one thing and that I could be a bit of a flibbertigibbet. But I took it as criticism, that I wasn't *able* to be good at anything. I wonder now if it was misdirected self-criticism; my mother trained as a chiropodist but never fulfilled her professional potential. She married at nineteen and immediately became a housewife and mother. She was a feisty Yorkshire woman and I can only imagine how diminished she felt at times. I'm accomplished in many areas, but her words still make me doubt myself. A mother's words cut deep.

With my peripatetic RAF background, in some ways airfields have always felt like home to me. My father's last posting found us living near Old Windsor, which is below the flight path of Heathrow. He and I became *those* people, the ones who stand on the top floor of Car Park 2 at Heathrow with airband radio and binoculars, watching the aircraft coming and going and listening to all the flight deck conversations. I remember running in from the family garden and announcing, 'There goes the 6pm Concorde to New York!'

After A-levels, I chose to study for a two-year bilingual secretarial course, six months of which involved working in Paris for the Ministry of Agriculture. I flew to Paris for the internship and a little spark was lit in me. I was captivated by the cabin crew – they looked so smart and I imagined how fabulous their job must be. A seed was sown somewhere in my brain. Although it was only a European flight, it seemed to me that they inhabited a marvellous world. I was on the cusp of adulthood and life was full of possibilities and places to go.

After college I got a job with Trans World Airlines and then British Airways as a ground agent at Heathrow. I was captivated by the thrill and workings of an international airport; it took me straight back to my feelings as a young girl on that first flight. We'd flown then as a family from Heathrow and it had lost none of its magic for me. Like the child I once was, poring over atlases and magazines and books about travel and foreign countries, I wanted to be part of this exciting place, full of aeroplanes, with the opportunity to travel to places like India and the Seychelles. The terminals were filled with people of different nationalities and they fascinated me. I was envious as I watched the flight and cabin crews walking through the terminal, looking so chic.

When I was twenty I joined Iran Air as cabin crew. I did my training in Dublin and Tehran and had a marvellous time making friends. It was fun and exciting all being thrown together, and it gave me rich insights into the lives of others because we were from such diverse backgrounds. It's hard to imagine now, but at that time to have friends from so many countries was in itself very unusual and exciting.

Eighteen months later the Shah of Iran was overthrown, heralding the Iranian revolution, and all non-Iranian employees were made redundant. I was relieved for myself, but worried for my Iranian colleagues living under the regime of Ayatollah Khomeini. After the revolution I worked for British Airways, the nation's flag carrier. In recent years we've come to see flying as just another form of transport, not very different from catching a train. In the late 1970s and early 80s, however, to be cabin crew was seen as prestigious and exciting. Competition for the job was stiff and many of my friends envied me. The uniform was expensive, elaborate and glamorous, and I was tremendously proud to wear it. I felt that I was working for the best airline in the country, if not the world.

But I didn't want to be cabin crew. I wanted to be a pilot. This was the late 1970s, when it was almost impossible for a woman to become a pilot. You needed to convince the airline that you were not only as good as, but much better than, the men. It was accepted thinking that training a woman was a waste of money because she'd just go off and have children. Many employers wouldn't even consider employing women for that reason. I didn't have the maths and physics background to apply, anyway – girls of my generation were often not given the opportunity to study maths and science. Subjects like that were not something we should worry our pretty little heads about. We were certainly not encouraged to take STEM subjects, as girls are today.

I had my daughter when I was thirty-one and returned to British Airways after my maternity leave. I really didn't want to give up my job, but I felt selfish and guilty leaving my little girl. I felt that I shouldn't be away enjoying myself. It's painful to think that there was no infrastructure to enable me to continue with the career I loved. I wanted to stay with British Airways and become a trainer for cabin crew or move into management, but we lived too far away from Heathrow for me to make the daily commute. We didn't have a discussion about the family moving closer to the airport in order that I could continue my career. It just didn't happen in those days. There was always the expectation that a woman's career would be secondary to that of her husband and that it was selfish to expect otherwise.

My mother died in 2012, the same year that I was diagnosed with endometrial cancer. I was fifty-five, and my world was turned upside down. I adored my mother – she was very loving. She was also forthright, matriarchal and critical. The combination of her death and my being ill became a transformational time for me. I wasn't answerable to her about my decisions anymore, and that was surprisingly freeing. Nobody knows how long we've got on this planet, and I think it focused my attention on *me*, possibly for the first time in my life. What did I want to do now?

These past few years I've been working on resolving this inner tension. I think I was afraid of failure, but I also knew that I could do better for myself. I've always been an assistant to someone and I've never put myself first. But the thought that 'I can do that!' has never gone away. Since my mother died I've started to push myself. I've studied for a BA and an MA and I've begun to find my voice. The younger me was only ever heard over the aircraft's PA system!

Being diagnosed with cancer was a huge shock and of course there were anxious months of treatment and waiting for test results, but it did focus my mind. I decided to start flying lessons as soon as I was well enough. I remember my first flight so clearly – it was 1st July 2018 when I slid into the left-hand seat of the single-prop, blue-and-white Piper Warrior, buckled up and put on my headphones and boom mike. It was a near perfect day, with a clear blue sky with only a few wisps of cloud above us. As Harry, the instructor, started to taxi us out, I glanced down at my family waving from the concrete apron below. Once on the runway, as instructed, I kept a light touch on the aircraft's dual control column to follow through on Harry's movements. It didn't take long to gain height to 2,500 feet above the English countryside. After decades of dreaming and disappointment and numerous hours of flying as cabin crew, I was, at last, learning to fly. This felt like the best journey of all.

Until the Covid lockdown in 2020, I was flying every fortnight if the weather allowed. The physics of flying aren't that difficult. I fly a Piper Warrior single-engine propellor aircraft. It's a basic machine; it has a fuselage and it has wings, so it will fly, provided you do a few basic things. It's all about balancing the opposing forces of weight versus lift and thrust versus drag. The basics aren't difficult: keeping the angle of the wing correct, flying at the right speed, and knowing what to do if the wind suddenly knocks you sideways. The plane is fairly forgiving as long as you almost let it do what it wants to do.

We fly under visual flight rules, which means flying in weather conditions clear enough to allow the pilot to see where she is going without the use of instruments. As this means you can only fly in daylight and in good weather you need to be flexible with your diary. I'm disappointed that I'm not closer to taking my first solo flight, but recently a lot of lessons have been 'spun' either because of poor weather or due to the many months that the flying school was closed during the pandemic. It's been frustrating, but I'm determined to get my Private Pilot's License (PPL). Flying is quite a big commitment. In some ways it's straightforward, with strict protocols and procedures to follow, but the mental and emotional rigour is hard – it tests you in every way because a silly mistake could cost you your life. I always go into the coffee shop after my flying lesson to write up notes about how I think the lesson went, about my thoughts and feelings, and what I need to focus on next. I don't think I'm fearful when I'm up there, but flying gives me a huge adrenalin buzz and it's important to spend some time in calm reflection.

To anyone who would like to learn to fly, I would strongly suggest they try an 'experience flight' to see if they feel comfortable in a small four-seater aircraft that sits just seven and a half feet off the ground. If you're nervous on that experience flight, then I think it's probably something you shouldn't pursue.

In terms of equipment and gear, you need remarkably little. You'll need headphones with a boom mike, and a set of manuals to accompany your study. You'll start in the briefing room with your instructor, who will tell you about the basics. You'll be given a checklist and then you'll probably do an hour's experience flight. The instructor will talk you through everything: walk you out to the aircraft, walk around the aircraft with you, and talk you through its every moving part. The student pilot sits in the left-hand seat (the seat that belongs to the pilot-in-command) with the instructor on the right. You must pass a medical examination before your first solo flight.

Most of the effort in learning to fly is mental. I've had to fight hard to change the rhetoric in my head. Rather than seeing myself as being selfish for doing this, I'm changing my attitude to being focused, determined and confident, in order to give myself energy. It's challenging after all my early conditioning. As well as the practical flying exams, there are nine ground school theory exams, each one of which has a hefty manual to study and commit to memory. It's easy to be blown off course to attend to the needs of family or other 'shoulds' and 'oughts' that are so well rehearsed.

I think part of wanting to fly is a rather belated feminist stand. I was prevented from – or at least not encouraged in – following my dreams. I'm now a member of the British Women Pilots' Association, which encourages women and girls into aviation. I want to support young women in realising their aspirations of becoming pilots and astronauts. We're making huge strides, but it's still not a level playing field. And women's equality can be pulled back overnight, just as it was at the end of World War II, when all the women pilots were required to return to roles as housewives and mothers to make way for the men to return.

I think it can be difficult for family members when their loved ones learn to fly. They may think we're amazing, but mostly they worry whether we're safe or taking unnecessary risks. And as in all relationships there can be feelings of jealousy and abandonment when a loved one finds a new interest. There is a reality to accept: people do have accidents and light aircraft do crash, even though the same can be said of so many things we do every day.

One of the life lessons I've learned from flying is that sometimes the wisest course of action is counter-intuitive. For example, if you get a warning light that your airspeed is dropping and there's a risk of getting into a stall, you should 'lower the nose' to pick up airspeed again. Instinct tells you to bring the nose up, but trying to climb and regain height isn't going to be helped by applying full throttle. The opposite will happen. It's important to take a breath, lower the nose and check that everything is working, that you are reading the instruments correctly, that the weather conditions are safe to be flying. That *you* are safe to be flying. That you are in balance. I'm trying to apply this principle to my own life. There's a profound space of healing to be found in retreating for a while – withdrawing from the noise and urgency of the world and taking time to hear yourself. This feels like an essential part of what it means to be a wise woman.

The realisation that being a commercial pilot can now never be a career for me fills me with regret. I wish I had the chance to live my life all over again. Nonetheless, I'm loving working towards getting my pilot's licence. For anyone out there who wants to learn to fly (or anything else, for that matter) – don't put obstacles in your own way. Don't spend forty years thinking about it. As my ninety-two-year-old father said to me, 'Do it, just do it! I have a little mantra in my head to help me safely pick up speed: 'Lower the nose; lower the nose.'

10

CAROLINE'S STORY: BACK IN THE PICTURE

There comes a point in each of our lives when we face a choice. Will we stay as we are, embracing the pale shadow of womanhood ... or will we sink deep into the heart of the bog, and find out what it is to reclaim our creative power as women.

Sharon Blackie, *If Women Rose Rooted*

Ledbury is my local town, and I am very fond of it. Its 17th-century black-and-white Market House, cobbled streets and timbered coaching inn give it a sense of timelessness. Ledbury celebrates its long association with poetry and poets – Elizabeth Barrett Browning, John Masefield, Rupert Brooke, Robert Frost and Edward Thomas to name but a few – with the annual International Poetry Festival. The town also prides itself on its independent shops and so I was excited when I saw that a new gallery, Take 4, had opened. While talking to Caroline, the owner, I discovered that she was a member of the choir I had just joined. We chatted every time I visited the gallery and I soon came to realise that she was a Juicy Crone, a woman making a new life in her third act. I felt confident that in this place of poets, writers and artists there was a lot for me to learn. Caroline and I have spent many a happy hour since, wrapped in coats and scarves, drinking cappuccinos alfresco at a local café, sharing our stories. Here she tells us about the road she took to opening Take 4, and how it changed her life completely.

So there I was, listening to Sir Roy Strong making his speech at the opening of my new venture, the Take 4 Gallery. He was dapper, as ever, in a velvet suit. His wasn't a cursory speech, but fulsome, genuine in his delight at opening a gallery in Ledbury. He emphasised the importance of art and culture in society, how essential it is to create a platform for art to thrive, and how passionately he felt the consequence of art in all its forms is for our well-being.

It was 28th March 2019, almost exactly forty years after I'd had to give up on my first degree in Fine Art. I couldn't have been prouder – or more overwhelmed – by what was happening. It would have been very easy to deny that this was about me, my passion, my adventure. Sir Roy raised his glass: he was toasting new beginnings, a place for artists to showcase their work and for would-be artists to learn to paint and draw. So was I, but I was also toasting friends and family who had advised, cautioned, supported, cheered and championed me to make this happen. Uncharacteristically – silently, inwardly – I was also toasting myself. The gallery represented so much to me: my sense of self, new beginnings, me starting a whole new chapter of my life.

It had been just a few weeks since I took on the lease of the little double-fronted, bow-windowed Georgian shop. My good friend Winona was there by my side, as she had been throughout this journey. Winona believed in me and the business – supporting me in every possible way. Ever since we viewed the property, I had been on cloud nine, and no amount of caution in the voices of my nearest and dearest could dampen my enthusiasm. Of course, they were absolutely right that I needed to write a business plan, that it was important to have projections for the coming year, and that I needed contingency money to guard against the unexpected. (How could I possibly have prepared for the events of March 2020?) I understood and accepted all of this, but this was about being me. I was undeterred.

I had always loved art; I studied History of Art at A-level and then went on to study for a Fine Art degree in Cheltenham. I love all aspects of art, but when I studied the history of art I found I was drawn to the artists' personal stories, to what made them tick and how they became the artists that they were. However, like many women of my era, I got married and became pregnant before I completed my degree. The college was prepared to let me finish the course with my baby in tow, but the logistics were impossible for me. I didn't feel I could give the time I needed to complete the course, especially given the intensity of the degree show, and anyway, learning to look after your firstborn is a full-time occupation in itself.

Yet here I was today, a sixty-something woman owning and opening my first business. I was on a high. All my life I'd wanted to be an artist, but after my first pregnancy I had three more children. I love them dearly, but four children take a lot of time and energy (and money) and it was almost impossible to carve out space for myself to draw or paint. Raising four children from birth through to leaving home spanned thirty years, and even now some of them keep bouncing back! Most of my creative energy went into encouraging and supporting my husband and family. I did a lot of art and craft with the children when they were small, but it was rare for my own creative urges to be met. I – and my creativity – needed time apart from the family, space to be in my own psyche. That's not something you can snatch for a few moments here and there. I didn't feel as if I had an identity of my own, because I was always doing something for everyone else.

There came a particularly dark time in my life when my father died. I was in my late forties, devastated by the loss, and found myself in the grip of serious depression and anxiety. We had a wonderful relationship, chatting on the phone most days. He had a great sense of humour and I enjoyed the banter between us. He was my go-to person. After his death I needed a lot of help, some of it in hospital. It was a really difficult time. Life became hard for me to understand, and through the depression I became more and more isolated. I'm not a loner, not the sort of artist who's happy to be squirreled away in a garret for days on end. I love meeting people and being with friends.

I remember one Christmas Day I felt so lost that I started looking for jobs, anything that caught my eye, on the internet. I think I was trying to find a healthier direction for myself. I knew somewhere deep down that I was a good artist and that that was what I needed to do. I listened too much to other people and I should have been stronger and listened to myself far more. I didn't find anything that day, but it was the start of me finding my way back to fulfilment.

The spark in me was rekindled after my third child started school. I took a part-time job in a nearby gallery. I absolutely loved it and started to sketch again while I was there. It seemed to tap into a vein deep within me and something started to flow. I began to think, to dream, to know that this was really what I wanted to do. But then I became pregnant with my fourth child and the baby became my focus. I lost my way again for a while.

Depression is a bleak state. One day my eldest son, Thom, who was thirty-one at the time, came home and found me crying. He drew a picture of me: the tears and I were draining down the plughole. He said, 'Mum, you're disappearing. You need to do art, you need to draw.' He was right. I started to draw again. Who was it who said that expression is the opposite of depression? It's certainly true in my case. It's almost as if I'd been denying myself the very essence of me, the thing that makes me who I am. Art is the expression of self for me. As soon as I got back to giving myself the time to draw and paint, things started to change.

Again, it was my son Thom who encouraged me, ten years ago, to study for an MA in Fine Art. This was such a gift to myself. I focused my work on the notion of chairs: empty chairs, manly chairs, chairs no longer occupied by family members, but still feeling their presence, chairs that faced away, where the voice of the occupant is not heard. It freed up so much in me – I'm now able to be more expressive and courageous. And as my confidence has grown, so has the size of the canvases I paint! I love setting up a huge canvas and capturing the essence of the Malvern Hills. It's a glorious landscape.

Coming to Ledbury in my late fifties after the MA was a springboard for change, the beginning of a new way of life for me, and my artwork began to take off. I found myself a studio. Virginia Woolf was right: we do need a room of our own. Having my own space altered my perception of this being my work, my profession – not just a hobby. As a mother of four I'm so used to being on call all the time that I'd forgotten that it's possible to be alone doing your own thing with no interruptions.

As well as making my own art again, I also started teaching art in a café and gallery. This was something I could give that also gave me a lot of joy. That began a small but regular stream of income, and I realised that perhaps this could become the reliable side of my business, and that, knowing I had a steady income, it might be possible to open a gallery. Teaching art also helped me to reconnect with people and diminished my feelings of isolation. Chatting with other people about art frees us up to talk about the bigger things in life – existential questions and shared vulnerabilities.

My confidence started to build, and I entered the Sky Arts *Landscape Artist of the Year* competition. On three occasions I was chosen from hundreds of entries for a 'wild card' place. You're given four hours to paint a landscape and, as if that isn't challenge enough, for one of these I was painting in oils in the pouring rain and the wind was so strong that the canvas blew right in my face. Nonetheless the judges' very positive comments as they wandered around gave me a huge boost. I also had a stall selling my art at the Countryfile Show at Blenheim Palace. Countryfile decided they would like to film me painting the palace and putting Winston Churchill and his dog in the foreground. It was a huge honour.

Gradually, I felt a shift inside me and my artwork started taking off. I began to realise that I had a lot to give. There was so much joy in this; I changed the way I thought about everything. Whereas before I'd had huge anxiety problems, I now knew that I had a practical way to resolve those feelings. It's really helped me.

I remember so well coming to view this property. Winona and I had looked at several other commercial outlets but nothing really 'spoke' to me. I heard on the grapevine that this building, which had been a children's clothing shop, was available to rent. It was a miserable January morning, and the building was cold and empty and looked rather sad. Despite this it felt exactly right. There was an area at the back for my studio, some storage cupboards, and a courtyard garden. The front of the shop, with two bay windows, was light and airy and spacious, with lots of walls for hanging art and room enough for a table to display three-dimensional works.

Securing the lease and moving in happened quite quickly. The first thing we did was cover up the windows while we set to on sprucing the place up. We laid a new floor and painted the walls grey, with lime green highlights that reflected the light beautifully. We refurbished an interesting old cabinet to display jewellery. Two days before the opening we took the paper screen down from the windows and gasped: we'd forgotten how wondrous the bay windows were. They were bigger than we remembered, perfect for displaying pottery and sculptures and for attracting customers in.

I decided to call the gallery Take 4. The philosophy is to showcase the work of local artists in at least four different mediums and to change the displays every six weeks. I like to have a variety of mediums such as paint, pen and ink drawings, photography, encaustic work, jewellery, ceramics and sculpture. Showcasing an artist's work is a big responsibility and of course there's risk involved, such as breakages and theft. Fortunately, I've had very few of those.

Selling art is not a predictable business and I had to accept from the start that I might see huge fluctuations in sales. It's very important to me not to have to worry about money, as that's a block to my creativity. Knowing that I can teach art classes to cover the rent gives me the psychological freedom to be my true creative self the rest of the time.

I love meeting people – they often chat as they look at the exhibitions. People are fascinating, and we learn so much from each other. Friends often put their head around the door to say hello as they go about their shopping. It's just what I'd hoped for – a hub of friendship. Shortly after I opened Take 4, I attended the first meeting of the Ledbury Traders Association. Winona warned me before I left not to volunteer for anything. So how I managed to return from that meeting as the newly elected chairperson, I don't know. Winona's loving response was a silent roll of her eyes, which I interpreted as 'you stupid woman!' I was completely inexperienced as a trader and had a lot to learn, but I was more than a little in love with Ledbury and believed that by looking at everything with fresh eyes I could contribute some good ideas.

During the first Covid lockdown of 2020, after four days spent sitting at home trying to find inspiration and not knowing how long my gallery would remain closed, I had the idea to make sketches for frontline workers as a little thank you to them. I posted an invitation on Facebook for nominations for key workers and others who might enjoy the gift of a pen-and-ink sketch of their pet. I did about forty sketches, and people told me how much they meant to them. I'm now turning them into greeting cards.

What took me so long to open my own gallery? Do I wish I'd done it earlier? In many ways I do, except it wouldn't have been possible where we were living at the time. We needed a change of location. I guess there's a natural order to everything and now certainly feels like the right time. Some people feel a decline in energy as they age, but with no caring responsibilities I feel energised, and I can put so much passion into the gallery. I love it – it doesn't feel like work. It's a joy. I did have practical experience of working in a cooperative and of helping in someone else's gallery, so I have a lot of knowledge and skills to bring to my own business, but I still have to pinch myself and tell myself that I've done this. I'm running a successful gallery. I'm not an imposter. That being said, opening my own gallery in my sixties feels very exciting and decidedly grown-up! It's also the fulfilment of a hidden longing. This represents so much more to me than the opening of a small business: it's about learning to be myself in my wisdom years.

Owning the gallery has given me an identity. I feel so different now. When I went through the period of deep depression, I lost my way. And even as I recovered, my identity had been so strongly enmeshed in family that I still lost sight of myself. When you have children you know exactly who you are. You know unequivocally where you're invested. When that goes, it can rock your foundation, and it's easy to feel that you are 'nothing'.

It's very easy for me to think that I haven't achieved this, that someone else has opened this gallery, someone who's doing a really good job. I still have to pinch myself and think: it's here, I've done this. Many people warned me of all the responsibilities, but it's not as onerous as you might think. It's manageable and oh, so rewarding.

My husband is proud of what I've done. He loved the launch night at Take 4 and often helps out in the gallery. I also know that if my father were alive, he would be thrilled. He would love this place and would get as much from coming here as I do. I sort of feel his presence. Fifteen years ago I could never have imagined having had such a meaningful few years as I have since I opened Take 4. Sir Roy was right: it has been central to my well-being. This is me. I hope too that, in some small way, those who come for art lessons, or who perhaps spend a little time enjoying the works on show, also feel that it has enhanced their lives.

11

GINNY'S STORY:

WALKING BESIDE YOU

Tell me, what is it you plan to do
with your one wild and precious life?

Mary Oliver, *The Summer Day*

I met Ginny very late on in the writing of this book. I was looking to step out into my new world and had booked a holiday to Norway with WalkingWomen – walking in the mountains with twelve women whom I had never met before, but who so rapidly became friends and trusted confidantes. As we shared stories, and much laughter, together, I gained insight, strength and hope. (I have decided there should be a new collective noun: a *wisdom* of women walking.)

I am honoured that Ginny shared her story with me and grateful too that she helped me get it 'beach-ready' so quickly! Her experience of personal loss allows us to reflect upon just how important it is to have women walking beside us, hearing our stories, encouraging our dreams; and how the act of 'walking by the side' of someone is both an honour and a gift. Ginny has bought and is developing an adventure travel company for women which not only embraces her ethical principles but also meets the needs of her newfound life.

On 5th September 2015, at exactly 7.41am, my life changed for ever. My partner took her last breath as we lay together in the home we had shared for over 20 years. The place where I had loved waking up each morning to share a coffee and chat about whatever was on our minds, or had been in our dreams. The place where we had laughed and loved and now I had lost. Today was a different day.

I wasn't alone. In the next room were two of my greatest friends. They lived down the road, but had chosen to stay the night as they felt Maggie had reached her last few days. They didn't want me to face this alone. I'm not sure what I would have done without them. I could already hear them on the phone calling our other friends and the house began filling with our nearest and dearest.

'What now?' I wondered. Where has Maggie gone? What do I do after two years of caring, of hospital visits, of travel, of parties and celebrations to live every moment of life to the full?

The future we had once imagined, gone.

My friends were Irish, and they came dressed in their best clothes out of respect. 'Sit still,' they said. We all had tea and sat with Maggie and just talked about the great life we had all had together, of what Maggie had given us. 'No rush.' This helped me in the days to come. 'No rush…'

Maggie left to the sound of *The Flower of Scotland*, her favourite Scottish anthem. She was Scottish and so proud to be. We raised a glass of whisky together, toasting her.

Then, the house was empty, so empty, but I knew I needed to be alone. I needed to just sit, no rush, and think and feel. What would come next, I wondered?

From the moment she died I wanted to live, but there were times when I thought it was just too hard. It was my darkest time ever. I sought help from a psychotherapist, who specialised in grief work. I would wake up in the mornings with no energy, I had no enthusiasm, I felt numb and didn't recognise myself. I wanted to live positively, I wanted to feel again. I do now, but it has taken me several years.

Through all that tragedy I had people who walked beside me that made it possible for me to journey on. People who came night and day to be there for me. Maggie didn't want many people around, just me, but that became intense. It was wonderful that friends dropped by to check that I was okay. She didn't want to die, but she died in her own bed, with her favourite music playing, with me beside her. And again, as her coffin left our home pulled by black horses, all our friends and family walked beside me, behind the coffin. My six closest women friends carried Maggie's coffin – it was such a powerful image, the strength of women supporting each other, holding each other up.

I think it helped everyone to feel they had a role. I am a resilient person, but I realise that I could not have done that alone. The friendships, which were already deep, became even stronger. These women continued to walk beside me. I had support from friends, family and colleagues, and I managed to keep getting up and moving, even though my heart was broken, and I was in the darkest place I had ever been. It was an unknown place for me – I've had the luxuries in life of a strong, supportive family, great friends, and a great love. I kept thinking: How has this happened to me?

Earlier, friends had advised me that I needed to keep an open mind about work. So, even though I had given up my job to spend precious moments with Maggie, I had kept some doors open. A charity I was doing some part-time work for had a CEO vacancy, and my friend, an ex-colleague, encouraged me to go for it. Personally I questioned how I could take on such a big role when my head was in a blur and I could hardly think straight. With support I applied, and I got the job.

A few days later, I found myself walking into the Beanstalk charity office in London to meet the team as the new CEO. I remember getting to the door of the office and thinking that I would not be able to walk through it. But I did, and for the next five years I ran the charity – there were many meltdown moments but, somehow, I managed. Once again it was due to the people by my side, the people who were always there to lift me up. I had lost confidence through my bereavement, but slowly, slowly, I started to re-emerge.

It wasn't just work that changed. I also knew I couldn't carry on living in the home that *was* Maggie and me. The home where she had lived and died. Everywhere I looked I saw her sick self – the medical equipment we had to have, the new furniture that meant she could be comfortable. I got rid of it swiftly, but I just couldn't get rid of the feelings. One night I realised that I needed somewhere new. I wasn't ready to sell up and leave this life, but I needed something, somewhere, that would give me fresh perspective. A special place I could holiday and get away.

Maggie and I had talked of buying a house somewhere warm. Somehow, I found myself looking at the website for the TV show *A Place in the Sun*. 'We are looking for house hunters', it said – and I applied. Unbelievably, the next day the phone rang. It was a researcher from the show who told me my application had arrived at just the right time and would my sister and I come to be interviewed to see if we were TV worthy? Help! I hadn't even told my sister I was doing it! 'Give me a few moments,' I replied, and I rang Sara. As always, she came to my aid and said she would come with me. She is my big sister, and she is always there for me.

Off we went to some recording studio on the outskirts of London and the next thing we knew we were being filmed for *A Place in the Sun*: *Home or Away*. We spent three days in Dorset and three days in the Costa Tropical. My main specification was that the house needed to be close to the sea – somewhere I could swim. I cried my way through the process, thinking how much Maggie would have laughed, how bizarre it all seemed. In Spain I found my dream house and immediately put in an offer. Casa Margarita has been my haven for the past five years – the place where I go to be alone, but also the place I go to holiday with family and friends to enjoy the warmth, the Spanish joy of life, and my beloved sea. The house has a view of the ocean and in just five minutes I can be in the water.

One morning as the sun rose I scattered some of Maggie's ashes there. And I wondered – would I sink or would I swim? Part of me wanted to float away, but the bigger part wanted to embrace life, embrace the new me and a life without my big love. Casa Margarita helped me renew my joie de vivre and from there new things began to happen.

Back in London, my CEO role was demanding. I felt I was losing energy, and the years of caring were taking their toll, so I decided I needed to take three months off to rest a little. My sister-in-law asked me if I might like to do the Mongol Rally, which her son had done a few years earlier. Not many women do it, but she thought we would make a good team. I knew that when I was with Saf we always laughed a lot. I also knew she wanted to get away, to really try something new and find out more about who she was.

In August 2018 we drove out of London on our way to Mongolia. We had driven a few miles when my phone went. It was my nephew telling me I had left my rucksack on the drive! No way could I turn back – we were on our way and there was no stopping us. Our Nissan Micra had enough stuff in it, and anyway I was travelling light.

Six weeks later we were in Ulaanbaatar, the capital of Mongolia, having driven across Poland, through the Baltic States and across Russia. A trip you couldn't do now, but we saw the best of Russia. Sitting beside my sister-in-law, driving through remote places, we talked and talked. It was such a wonderful adventure and once again I was reminded of the power of friendship. I felt honoured that she wanted to do this with me. It transpired that we both had things to talk about and side by side in a car for six weeks we talked and talked, cried and laughed our heads off. We had so many hilarious moments.

After completing the epic rally I realised that I needed more in my life, and that I wanted travel and adventure to be at the heart of whatever came next. Friends kept telling me about 'WalkingWomen', group activity holidays for women, but I couldn't quite take the plunge. Maggie and I had always loved holidays – not in groups, but just us. It was our time to be together. How do you holiday without a partner? To be among strangers and in groups was not my thing. I think I had lost confidence about being with people. I was also adjusting to being single. A friend said, 'Don't think of meeting people as being about dating, or finding a partner – it's just about being curious about other people and meeting new friends.' Slowly I emerged, feeling curious… I didn't want to do 'groupy' things, but then I'd started to do things with 'coupled' friends and I didn't always want to do that either! Eventually, after years of friends pointing me towards WalkingWomen holidays,

I decided to investigate. Perhaps a new place and a new activity, bringing new memories, would be good. I decided to give the cross-country skiing trip to Norway a go. I had never tried cross-country skiing, and I had never been to Norway. I do, however, have an affinity with snow. I was born in January in 1963, the worst winter on record, and my mum always tells me the story of how she had to wrap me up tight as it was so cold – I love the image of being born in a blizzard!

So, off I went, and I haven't looked back. The guide was so welcoming and supportive. The group of women all had their stories, but each of them was there to be active, experience something new and try and spot a moose! I felt so energised being in the company of these lively, enthusiastic, fun women. Without a partner I found I was still able to find real intimacies and adventurers to share experiences with. Slowly, slowly I was emerging. No rush… Something about the landscape in Norway changed my outlook. It was expansive, and I think in some strange way that enabled my feelings to be similarly expansive. I went with no expectations; I didn't feel I needed new or more friends. However, I returned believing that I did have room for more people, new friends in my life.

And then, in March 2020, around the time my sister turned sixty, Covid appeared. Travel ground to a halt and I was thrust into living alone. Luckily a friend was moving to the US, and, in a flurry, I found myself moving into her house on the Thames – close to friends and near my sister. I realised I really needed company and also that I needed to change my life, to do something different. I felt I needed space away from London. Everywhere I walked in the city reminded me of Maggie's sick days. Where we lived, and now where I worked, was right next to the hospital, where we spent so many hours for her chemotherapy and consultations. I was tired of facing it every day. I needed somewhere new and something fresh. I also wanted to be free of a mortgage and give myself more possibilities.

I gave up my CEO role, after taking the charity to a new home in a bigger charity, and I sold the London flat that had been my home with Maggie for over 20 years. I went summer hiking with a friend I had met a few years earlier. At our first meet she asked me 'How can I help you?' and from then on she became the person who invited me to new things and helped me build my confidence to jump into more new things. Again I felt the power of women's friendship. What a difference it can make to have someone there for you.

It was this friend who introduced me to another hiker... A woman who I felt I wanted to walk beside, who I wanted to talk to, who I was curious about. I hadn't felt this for over five years. I think the selling of my London home, my past life, prepared me for opening my heart to new possibilities. Slowly, slowly, no rush – I gradually stepped into a new relationship. A relationship that takes us between Switzerland and Surrey as we share each other's lives. I have hope and love again. No rush...

I started to reflect on the nature of relationships. What is special about your significant person? Your big love? It's having someone walk beside you, with you; someone who has your back, who you know you can trust, who is there for you day in and day out. When that went, when Maggie died, I came to realise that I *could* find those things in other ways. It's not the same – you are not sharing a bed every night. But significant people had stepped up for me and were 'walking with me', side by side.

During lockdown, WalkingWomen came up for sale and I couldn't get it out of my mind. I reached out to talk to the owner, to express an interest and to ask about its philosophy – for her it was about giving women support, the space to be active and time to be in nature. It was about providing a safe, positive environment. Once again, I asked my sister to help and join me. Of course, she said yes!

I wanted to change how I worked. I knew I needed flexibility; I had always wanted to be an entrepreneur. And now I could have the freedom, with my sister, to make our own decisions – the freedom to shape WalkingWomen as we wanted to, with as little bureaucracy as possible. I needed an adventure, but I also wanted to be able to give back. This was not about making money; it was about offering women the chance to walk side by side together and support each other in the ways in which I had been so fortunate. And, if not now, when?

In August 2021, my sister Sara and I became the owners of WalkingWomen. It's a new venture for both of us and one that we are passionate about. We feel proud that we can continue a company that was founded to provide great walking holidays for women. We started running holidays in February 2022 and six months later had run fifteen holidays and notched up more than 150 bookings for the year. We continue to offer classic WalkingWomen holidays that have always been popular – to Glaramara in the Lake District, to Snowdonia, to Yorkshire and, my old favourite, Norway. We have city breaks in Newcastle and Copenhagen. But we have also introduced new places that mean something to us – Andalucia, which I now call home; Switzerland, which has brought me such joy; and Ireland, where I used to live.

WalkingWomen offers women the chance to find their 'tribe', role models who are adventuring and out exploring in nature. But just as important for most women is the sense of a safe place, where they can feel secure and supported. We have several levels of difficulty on offer, from gentle strolls to rigorous mountain hikes. But it's not about getting to the top as fast as we can; no-one is rushing. It's about kindness, and we all help each other along – we go at the pace of the slowest and if anyone needs an adrenaline fix they can run up and back down and re-join the group! We are mountain tortoises, but we *do* get to the top and we enjoy the view together. No-one is judging – you can be whoever you want to be. Everyone has a story to tell and needs that story to be honoured. Everyone is helped by having someone by their side when they need it. Having said that, we may have serious conversations as we walk, but we also have loads of fun, lots of laughter and a lightness of being. Play is important, no matter how old you are!

We have wonderfully loyal women guides, who we couldn't have got going without, and local partners in other countries keen to help us. We have also discovered the love so many women have for WalkingWomen. We have received so many calls to say well done and thank you for taking it on. So many loyal WalkingWomen followers are booking holidays, so many subscribe to our newsletter to hear more and so many are ready to share stories of their holiday experiences. One couple, returning to a WalkingWomen holiday in the Lake District, are coming from the US to spend their ten-year anniversary at a place that holds special memories for them. This year I met a seventy-one-year-old woman in Norway who had returned because she trusted WalkingWomen and wanted to regain her cross-country ski legs after being off the snow for thirty years. It's so heart-warming.

One thing we are keen to do is build up or 'be beside' women who are offering complementary skills such as writing, photography, cinematography or painting. We are also developing a partner page that lists female entrepreneurs and makers creating everything from comfortable underwear to outdoor gear. We use female guides and when we run our holidays overseas, whenever we can, we partner with trekking and hiking companies led by dynamic, adventuring women. Our bank is Starling Bank, founded by Anne Boden who is now the CEO.

Running WalkingWomen with my sister has energised me and given me a new way of life, one that at fifty-nine I am absolutely certain is right for me. I have the travel and flexibility I wanted and it has brought me the greatest adventure of all – which is to explore love again…

12

DEBORAH'S STORY: LAUGHTER REALLY IS THE BEST MEDICINE

Of course, to forget the past is to lose the sense of loss that is also memory of an absent richness and a set of clues to navigate the present by; the art is not one of forgetting but letting go. And when everything else is gone, you can be rich in loss.

Rebecca Solnit, *A Field Guide to Getting Lost*

Distracted by something, we have all missed our turning at one time or another. But as her husband drove around the roundabout for the third time, Deborah knew that her worst fears were playing out into their lives. They had passed all the other possible exit routes and only one remained. It was a terrible, pot-holed road, one that no-one, ever, should have to take.

When Deborah and I first met up it was a wet, muddy and bone-chillingly cold December day. We soon gave up on our plans to walk together and instead took refuge in my van. I had loaded it with blankets, hot-water bottles and flasks of coffee, as cafés were still closed due to the pandemic. Luckily the back seat is two metres from the front and with the sliding door open and all the windows down we were offered a little protection from the worst of the weather. As we talked, Deborah's painful story seemed to mirror those cold, dark days.

In April 2022 we met for the second interview for this project. In complete contrast, it was a bright, fresh spring day, perfect for wandering through water meadows filled with snake's-head fritillaries, cowslips and bluebells. The day reflected our mood entirely. We were both lighter than during our first meeting, daring even to laugh together, smile and enjoy the sunshine. Deborah had been through so much since our first meeting in 2020, and as she told me of her emerging plans for her new life the sense of regeneration and new beginnings was profound.

He snapped at me, 'Well it's dark! It's easy to get confused.'
I thought, but did not retort, 'This has been your route home from work for the last twenty years. How could you *not* know what exit to take?'

We made it home in silence. Each in our different and diverging worlds knowing what this meant, both grieving for a life that was disappearing and a future that was too awful to think about. In the few seconds it took to miss that turning, the minute and the hour of our fate became apparent. My suspicions had been confirmed.

I'd been worried about our relationship for some time. Atherton had been 'off' with me, he didn't seem particularly interested in what I was doing, nor keen to do anything with me. He didn't want to do the things we usually enjoyed together – not even a pub lunch, a concert, or even a walk. He ceased initiating anything and came over as distant. I didn't realise why and, given that the simplest explanation is usually the truth, I assumed it was about 'us'. I started to think we might be one of those couples whose marriage wouldn't survive retirement. I never imagined it was because he had dementia – why would I?

I recall that while on our first trip together as a young couple in Mexico, the ceiling fell in over breakfast. It was one of those relationship-defining moments. Were we to be outraged that it had happened or gleeful to have been spared? This time we weren't so lucky. Our lives were devastated by the weight of collapse.

Atherton was a consultant haematologist; I was the doctor's wife and his infrastructure. I was the provider of meals, clean sheets and clean shirts. I brought up our children. I paid the bills. I kept the house going, I managed the garden, sorted out the cars – whatever needed doing, I did it. He was free to pursue his career while I worked part-time as a freelance cookery book editor and writer. He was often on call and so I was used to being a 'single parent' at the drop of a hat. The phone could ring at any time, day or night, and his top priority was always the work. And of course, I could never get cross – if it was the maternity unit ringing after a difficult delivery, or A and E needing a consultation; we all expect our doctors to be there in an emergency – but of course it meant that I had to be available for everything the children needed. I don't regret a moment of it, because my children had a loving, secure home life and they have turned out as well-adjusted, lovely human beings, with good values, and I am dead proud of them.

Atherton reduced his working hours to three days a week when he was sixty, then fully retired at sixty-two. This was our time to have some freedom and fun together, or so we'd thought. We were at our best as a couple when travelling – he made me feel excited and alive. Our shared love of landscapes and cultures bound us and there was nothing we enjoyed more than trying to get to the heart of a place, discussing it over a cold beer on a sunny terrace. We always travelled lightly – although disproportionately heavy in medicines and first-aid equipment. However dangerous the trip, he made me feel safe. This enabled us to go to risky places such as the Lybian Sahara and the Amazon River; we rode trains through India; we even got to Tibet back in the day. We planned to use our new-found time to tick other places off our wish list.

This was not to be. Atherton's diagnosis of early-onset dementia turned me from a wife into a carer, and then the time came when his needs were too onerous for me to handle alone. The constant worry of where he was and what he was doing, the nighttime disruption, the consequences of the deterioration in his spatial awareness and his inability to manage his own needs, and then managing the incontinence, left me a shell of my former self. When the time came to transfer him to a care home in 2019, it was, honestly, the worst day of my life. The next day I had to begin the process of starting over as a single woman. That's hard when you still love your partner and long to be doing things with the person he used to be.

Before my marriage and up until the time the children were small, I had always lived in cities: Birmingham, London, Los Angeles. I had been a managing editor for a publisher. Rural life had taken some adjusting to, and I missed the buzz of urban life. So one of the questions I now faced was – where to live? Was I still at heart a city girl or was I now a country lass? The truth, I realised, was likely somewhere in between. Living in a small Wiltshire town probably suits me, mainly because this is where my friends are. I came to understand the value of friendship during Atherton's decline.

If I'm lucky, I told myself, I should have many good and active years ahead of me. How would I choose to spend this time and who was I going to be on this solo venture? Even thinking of going off and enjoying myself, knowing that my husband was in a care home, was a personal struggle. I don't think it's something you can resolve. Like so many women of my age, I had taken second place for so long that it's taking me time to explore that question – who am I going to be? – with integrity, to find answers that resonate. The question is existential. The answers might sound simple, but they come after profound negotiation, and not a little painful internal dialogue.

I have sought help from a variety of places, from talking therapy to yoga to Ayurvedic massage. Going back to university and studying for an MA in Creative Writing was probably the best decision I made. Not only was the writing cathartic, but I made a new group of friends, and it was entirely 'mine'. It became part of the 'I' that I was becoming.

Atherton always expected me to be strong and capable. He encouraged me to serve the community – to become a school governor and to get involved with local events. I felt the weight of this expectation and immediately got involved with campaigning for the Alzheimer's Society, in part because I know it is exactly what he would have imagined I would do in response to our situation.

Ours became a campaigning family for the Alzheimer's Society. Together with my two adult children, we went to the Houses of Parliament to lobby for improved funding of Alzheimer's in care homes. If Atherton had had another disease, such as liver failure or a stroke, the cost of his care would have been covered by the NHS – but Alzheimer's is not recognised for funding purposes. The cost of care is another burden to families already struggling to cope with a family member with dementia. Families are faced with bills of around £52,000 per annum, often much more – many people are wiped out of their savings within months. I was fifty-five when Atherton was diagnosed and there was a real possibility I would have to sell my home to pay for his care. The Alzheimer's Society made a video based on Atherton's and my experience, which went out on social media – my words are voiced by Lesley Manville. I like the idea of her playing me!

Maybe the scariest thing I have ever done in my life was to give evidence, via Zoom, to the Select Committee on Health and Social Care chaired by Jeremy Hunt in the House of Commons in July 2020. So nervous was I that a friend asked a speech coach to give me a pro bono session the day before! He taught me some of the tricks of the trade. That really helped and I felt I gave a confident and persuasive performance; it was good to make my voice heard on the injustice meted out to Alzheimer's patients and their families and to advise the government of what was needed to support us and signpost us to avenues of help. I grew more than a little that day and felt really empowered by advocating for myself and others, families who had also been dealt a difficult hand. This was the start of me finding my voice.

Atherton was a brilliant, talented man, with many interests – including writing prize-winning poetry. In 2017, not long after his diagnosis, he was still able to write a moving piece describing his loss of consciousness and sense of his historical self. It was heartbreaking to watch his decline. Within a few months, he became frail and soon little was left of the man I loved. His memories of our adventure-filled life together were gone, but I will treasure them forever.

There has been a tendency to sanctify Atherton, not just by me but by our children and family and friends. It's easy to forget that, lovely though he was and clever as he was, he too was human, fallible and not perfect. A husband who gifted me so much that I can take on my onward journey. However, I think I have always been in his shadow; it always felt a bit like 'and Deborah came too'. Perhaps recognising these feelings is part of the uncoupling. This is my time to step out and enjoy being me, whatever that means.

In many ways my husband died twice – the first time when I finally accepted that this brilliant man who I adored was just the essence of who he once was. And now that he has died, in the usually accepted sense, just three years later, this is another kind of bereavement. My children feel the same. I don't think we were expecting to grieve as much as we have. I thought I had grieved for him, and for us as a couple, when the Alzheimer's took him from me. I thought I had processed the tragedy as it unveiled, but that has not been the case. I am grieving all over again and sometimes it besieges me. I've spent a lot of time in the wee hours wondering how I can break free of the burden of expectation, and I think that may have contributed to experiencing his death a second time. Now he is no longer here I am trying to make my own decisions without feeling I am betraying him or being unfaithful.

Atherton always encouraged me to be independent throughout our marriage and I would go off on trips alone or with my girlfriends. Standing at an airport with a passport, on my own, had once been my idea of heaven – yet now doing this same thing, not out of choice but because he is no longer here, felt so different, as if I had lost a wing. There's no longer a partner back home to text and say, 'arrived safely', no-one to share stories with on returning.

One of the things I always wanted to do was to learn to scuba dive. After the agony of accepting that Atherton needed full-time care, I decided to take lessons on the small island of Cozumel, south of Cancun in Mexico. Those warm, turquoise Caribbean waters were the perfect place for me to learn – to take my first steps into my new life. I tried to remember the breathing I had learned in yoga, to keep it calm and even. My instructor helped me build skills and confidence until we were able to potter around the reef together, where she pointed out the huge variety of plants swaying under the water and the sapphire blue chromis fish darting about. A shoal of sergeant major damselfish glowed as they passed me and I saw my first angel fish. I was proud and excited by this first dive out. I decided I wanted to adventure more, both below and above water, and went on to get my PADI open-water diving certificate.

I felt too young to 'retire', but also, being freelance, I hadn't had a 'proper job' to retire from. I wanted to come out of the shadows, to admit that I still wanted a working life, to reclaim lost time. I am now writing for myself, starting to inhabit the persona of a single, freelance writer, which I find so much more gratifying than editing other people's work. I have had articles published in *Good Housekeeping*, *Living* and *Planet Mindful*. Following the publication of a piece in *National Geographic* about a couple of feminist cheese-makers in Mexico City, plus a slice of serendipity, I've been appointed as a judge for the 2022 World Cheese awards in Newport, Wales in November. I'm on a cheese roll you might say!

Last summer I went for a very early morning swim at Kemble, the source of the River Thames, as part of a writing workshop. My thoughts turned to Tamesis – the goddess or female spirit of the source of the river. I was with a group of like-minded women and I enjoyed the powerful feelings that came over the group – of beginnings and being in the 'source' of this mighty river. There was more than a little sense of conception and birth about that dawn swim. This summer I am also taking part in a re-enactment of the 350th anniversary of the Malmesbury witch trials. I'm really looking forward to getting dressed up as a witch and embracing my 'witchyness'; I fancy being 'up to no good' and throwing out a few hexes.

Three months after his death, I organised Atherton's secular memorial service. Everyone I loved and cared about was there. Although it was terribly sad, I enjoyed making all the arrangements, choosing the readings and shaping the occasion. I also wrote and delivered the eulogy; I was quite surprised and affected by how natural it felt for me to deliver the address. I found myself standing taller – I was comfortable in this role. I thought: I'm almost enjoying this. Someone said to me, 'It seems like you are coming out from under his shadow.' That made me cross, but I think there was more than a grain of truth in it, and I have reflected since on their words.

I am becoming much surer of who am in my own right and I feel a lot more comfortable in my own skin than I did a few years ago, but I also need to keep a little protective armour about myself. I don't know the shape of my future, but I'm determined to have fun discovering it. I feel like a frog on a lily pad. I'm wanting to leap, but the next pad isn't quite in sight yet – or else I'm not sure if it's a pad or just some weed! I suppose it will take time to know the difference.

It's funny, I used to have a lot of long hair, which I think I used to hide under. I also dyed it for appearance's sake. Then I found a really good hairdresser to give me a Jamie Lee Curtis-style pixie cut and, like her, I've let the grey grow in. I feel different with this new hairstyle, not worrying about what other people think

– slightly naughty and a bit sassy, with bright lipstick. It's a new take-it-or-leave-it me. People have enquired, out of interest, whether I want a new partner. I'm not looking for one, but I don't rule it out. Sometimes I long to be held, to be cherished and, yes, to feel that frisson of excitement again. Mostly, I want to smile and laugh and be lighter.

To that end, I decided to book myself on a comedy-writing course with Tony Hawks on the Greek island of Skyros. When I arrived, I didn't think the group looked like 'my tribe' and wondered what I was doing there. We were given some very silly things to do and there was so much fun and laughter that very quickly I lost my inhibitions. It was wonderful to unleash my funny side, to have a good belly laugh, to start to crack jokes – there's a real joy and reward in giving other people cause to laugh. I loved the feedback loop from that. It was wonderful to feel playful and, yes, youthful, after all the sadness. Holding an audience and making them laugh was a brand-new experience, one that really excited and empowered me. And I discovered that, after all, this *was* my tribe – we all felt safe enough as a group within a few days to go skinny-dipping in the moonlit sea together.

The Skyros course led me to drop into a 'yoga laughter' retreat in London for an article that I was writing. There I learned about the physiological effects of laughter, which has immediate effects on both the mind and body. It is a cliché but laughter is medicine – it relieves stress and helps us relax, stimulates our heart, lungs and muscles by taking in more oxygen-rich air, which in turn can lower our blood pressure. When we laugh our brains are washed with serotonin and dopamine, which make us feel better and more optimistic. Laughter can improve our immune system and relieve pain and help us cope with difficult situations. People who laugh recover more quickly from illness and those with chronic conditions report fewer relapses. The other brilliant news is that 'fake-it-till-you-make-it' works, too: the brain cannot tell the difference between real and pretend laughter. And perhaps most importantly of all, laughter connects us with other people, creating unity, sometimes in adversity.

After being with the yoga laughter group for just an hour, I felt like I was on drugs! We did a lot of role play, which sounds cringe-making but actually, being stupid in a group, laughing together about imagined scenarios and just being very silly, turned the laughter from contrived 'ha, ha, ha!', to real rippling belly laughter. Even now, telling you about it makes me smile and laugh. We all need to prescribe ourselves more laughter!

My recent experiences have pointed me towards continuing to find my voice, whether that is through writing or comedy or talking from the heart with friends. I want to explore the part of me that enjoys making people laugh, so I've signed up to go back to Greece. This time I might try a stand-up comedy workshop, venturing out of my comfort zone.

Who knows what else I will discover about myself?

13

JANETTE'S STORY:

I AM

You were once wild here. Don't let them tame you.

Isadora Duncan, *Isadora Speaks: Writings*
& Speeches of Isadora Duncan

Janette is the only woman in this book who has written her own story rather than work with me to create it from our interviews. It thus has a slightly different feel to the others. Janette was among those who spotted my call for Crones in Bradt's e-zine, and we met via Zoom. Life was restricted by the Covid pandemic and it was unlikely that we would meet in person any time soon. Despite living thousands of miles apart, we soon discovered we had a great deal in common. Like me, she felt her childhood had 'squelched' (silenced) her. She told me that as a child and an adult she struggled with an extra-sensory awareness, a psychic facility that never – until now – felt like a gift. Janette also honoured me with a story of her mother's love of early mornings – and how she would welcome them with the saying 'The day is not yet made.' The idea that every dawn holds the promise of new beginnings, of directing our own destiny and embracing our relationship with our flaws, is integral to the journey to Juicy Cronehood.

I feel so lucky to have met Janette, which would not have happened if my plan A for writing this book had worked out. Our friendship has grown beyond the scope of the project. We have been there for each other during this, the strangest of times, and despite an ocean between us, we have laughed together, cried together and held each other through stormy waters. We plan to celebrate our sixty-fifth birthdays together in the UK.

A tiny, wild girl-child sleepwalked into the world and found company there, in the trees and the hills and grass, and in the sheep, and the cows and dogs and cats and horses, and even the ants, and in all the other animals that were not as wild as she was, because they had been in the world much longer. The girl-child opened her mouth and yawned herself awake, and to her astonishment a low voice tumbled out. She talked to the animals, and they listened. Although they had not been tamed, they were less wild and less astonished than she was because they had grown used to the ways of the world, and to human beings being in the world, too. The girl-child opened her mouth and said the names of the animals, and they answered.

There were all kinds of humans in the world – gentle, quiet, loving ones, friendly and funny ones, and some with strange stares and loud voices. The animals had soft, animal voices and walked in their soft animal way, leaving no disturbance on the air. But the humans were loud, and the girl-child grew quiet as their noise grew louder, until it filled her ears and her eyes and even her mouth, and one day she choked on the loudness. She became silent and still then, and was lost inside silence for a long time. The animals kept vigil, and the trees and the hills and grass waited for her voice and her footsteps to return.

At last the girl stirred, and as she yawned herself awake, to her astonishment her voice tumbled out. She talked to the animals, to the dogs and the horses, and even the ants. She told them a story, and the animals told stories too – of their joys, and their aches and their fears. Their vigil was over because the girl was safe with them. They were untamed but not wild – not to her, and she was untamed but not wild – not to them. She learned to use her ears to muffle the loud voices, and allow others into her heart. She learned to see noise coming, like bright, coloured lights, and she kept out of the way of the harsh, gaudy ones and let only the soft ones in. She stayed close to the trees and the animals, to the dogs and the horses, and even the ants.

The girl grew curious about the story she was telling – a story that seemed to have no ending – and she set out on an expedition to discover where stories grow. She left the trees and the hills and grass behind, and made a promise to return. And a maybe can be broken, she told them, but a promise, never. The trees and the hills and grass, and the sheep, and the cows and dogs and cats and horses, and even the ants, and all the other animals, kept vigil.

I was raised on a smallholding in the wilds of Yorkshire, with a herd of Jersey cows, a trusty beagle hound, and two sheep and their lambs. There was a goat called Betsy, a flock of hens, a flurry of cats and kittens, and a neighbour's horse grazing in the home field. These were the sounds and companions of my childhood. Our ancient, rambling house stood on the hem of a tiny village, and was built of thick stone and was cold inside, in spite of the fire that always burned in the big kitchen. But this was home, where the morning milk was warm cream, and the eggs always fresh, and where sometimes a baby lamb lay in front of the fire, with the cats and the dog.

When I wasn't at play with the sheep and the dog, or exploring the hills with my two older sisters, I wrote poems and tiny stories, and letters to my parents. My mother said I was a 'fey' child, and had appeared, one day, out of nowhere. I was too young to understand; I thought it meant I was an interloper, but I think she meant I was mysterious, unworldly, supernatural even. My pale hair made me different from my raven-haired sisters, and I was tiny, with a deep voice and a crooked left eyebrow that someone named my 'evil eyebrow'. It was hard to belong among people. I stayed close to the animals and kept writing my poems. My mother kept all of my writings forever, especially one crumpled, small note that said:

Dear Mummy and Daddy. When I grow up I will always live near you.

After a decade my sisters and I were taken to the Netherlands, my father's home country. The sheep and the cows went away, and our cats, but the trusty beagle hound came with us. My sisters and I lived with our aunt – a loving and mischievous other-mother – in a beautiful warm house just a stone's throw from the palace in Soestdijk, while my parents built us a new home in a northern province. After a few years we returned to England, which never felt the same again.

As a girl I always felt as if I were reciting lines, as if life were a stage play or a poem. I could not make mistakes because then the whole story would cease to make sense, and everything would fall apart. I could hear in my head just how the lines should sound, and kept starting again from the beginning to make it perfect. It was hard work, and tiring, and eventually I stopped trying. I let other people speak for me, and I was sad but relieved. In her essay 'The White Album', Joan Didion wrote, 'I was supposed to have a script, and had mislaid it. I was supposed to hear cues...', describing a period in her life as:

> ...an adequate enough performance, as improvisations go. The only problem was that my entire education, everything I had ever been told or had told myself, insisted that the production was never meant to be improvised.

For much of my life I felt the way Didion felt. I couldn't find my script. It was safer to talk to a sheet of paper, where I could redact, or edit myself, in the privacy of the pages. When I learned that this painstaking, punishing process was just part of Becoming A Writer, and was being made much harder by Obsessive Compulsive Disorder, I trusted the process to unfold. I was sorely challenged, though, by strange contortions of my left thumb and fingers, and contortions in my left jaw and eye. I knew that it didn't look pretty but I could do nothing to stop it. It was not until I was forty that I learned I'd had Tourette Syndrome all my life. Somebody said, 'Well, it's a good thing you're nice looking, because the tics are really disfiguring.'

For a long time I hid. But life coaxed me out of the cupboard; I had poems and stories to write – even if my lines weren't pitch perfect. When I step up to the podium to read my work, the tics disappear. They simply melt away. Being in a state of flow, of profound concentration and absorption, can provide a temporary, palliative 'cure' for Tourette Syndrome. Sadly, the awareness that my face will be fleetingly, repeatedly disfigured causes stress of an opposite and more than equal force. Sometimes the tics in my thumbs grow so intense that I wear a hand brace. There's not much to be done for the jaw and eye tics other than heavy medications, which my body has become habituated to and are no longer effective. My jaw grinds and cramps, and the deepest relief is in sleep. And in writing. I wish I had known sooner that I have Tourette Syndrome; it might not have changed much, but knowing that it is a neurological disorder and not just weirdness makes it a little less stigmatising.

I went to college in the middle of England, in Staffordshire, where my parents moved when we returned from the Netherlands. I learned to love it for the beauty of its countryside and for the exquisite teacups that emerged from the labour of its smoky cities, but Staffordshire never was home. At college I met a young travelling man, a sailor, who by coincidence was of Dutch ancestry and had a Dutch surname. He told me stories of bold teenage adventures in South America, and I was inspired to keep him close. When our studies were complete we eloped to the West Indies, where we lived for almost a decade on a tiny island that I began to call home. In time, my parents forgave me for no longer living near them.

We went exploring together, the young man and I, and settled for a while on the island of Tortola in the British Virgin Islands. I taught French at a charter school and wrote columns about carnivals for the newspaper, and we settled in a lofty wooden house called Pelican Cliff House, cantilevered over a cliff, the waves crashing below us. We stayed there a long time and I practised belonging until it, too, became stormy. In 1989, Hurricane Hugo descended on the island and blew our house down. We retrieved from the surrounding hillside some belongings – rain-soaked, blue airmail letters and stained, precious travel books. The next months were spent moving from one house to another. Other people felt uprooted too, and it was a watershed period for many. After a decade of exotic, stormy travel and with our first child in my belly, we decided that my husband's business could support us all, and went to live in New England.

Our new home of Newport – on another tiny island, Aquidneck – was a friendly and manageable little metropolis with an international sensibility and a grassroots heart that welcomed us in. We had already been romanced by New England's white mountains and pristine villages, its weathered shingle and clapboard houses. It was an easy place to be, and I in turn embraced Newport, walking for miles with my baby son, exploring quaint colonial streets and sudden green parks. I kicked up the blossoms and leaves on the sidewalks as spring turned to summer, and summer and fall turned to the first biting, breathtakingly cold, winter. Our younger son was born three and a half years later, and our human family was complete.

I loved everything about motherhood. I embraced every whit of it. I experienced both my pregnancies as a state of grace; for nine months I was invincible, blooming, fecund, resplendent, protected in some altered, exalted state. Mothering came naturally to me, the love and the trials in it, and eventually my sons became my friends and sometimes, today, even my protectors and no longer my tiny charges to watch over.

As our boys grew we took them travelling far and near, to Kathmandu and the Grand Canyon, to Disney World and the Egyptian desert. On one of our 'near' adventures I was bitten by a deer tick. Weeks later, our sweetly coordinated family routine was turned inside out. I had contracted Lyme disease and two other infections, and would be living with the pain and fallout for the next eight years of my children's life. I pried the tick from my leg and took it to my doctor, where a nurse-practitioner tossed it the bin and pronounced that I was fine. 'Not to worry!' she told me. I researched my symptoms and knew I had Lyme disease, but it took four years to receive the diagnosis. I dragged my spent body from doctor to doctor. I was talked at but not listened to.

I was told I had multiple sclerosis, and then reassured it was just early menopause. Antidepressants would help. I was forty-four, and I was not menopausal. Months earlier I had been vigorous, robust and intellectually alert, writing poetry and giving readings. I wanted, humbly and passionately, just to mother my sons, teach, and study for a master's degree and a doctorate in poetry. In the office of the third doctor I consulted, I wept with frustration, with the pain, and from the weakness that kept me from walking on the beach with my dog; she patted my knee and said: 'There, there. Are your antidepressants working for you?'

One day, I stood at the kitchen window with the telephone in my hand and dialled my way down a long list of doctors in the hope of finding one – just one – who would really *see* me and hear my story. Each doctor was fully booked. The eighth doctor had a three-month waiting list, and I broke down, wept into the telephone, and garbled out my story. The receptionist was quiet and asked me to hold the line. Minutes later, she said, 'Dr Lanna can see you next week,' and I wept again, with gratitude and relief. Three weeks later, the doctor telephoned me with test results and said, 'I apologise on behalf of my colleagues in the medical profession. I don't know what they've been doing. You deserve better than this.' She confirmed Lyme disease with co-infections. 'It's been rocking and rolling inside you for years,' she told me. Her compassion and directness, and the relief of hearing the diagnosis, gave me the will to take charge again.

I kept my own medical records and insisted – when a treatment protocol felt wrong – that while the doctor was the medical expert, I was the expert of *me*. I chose to not fight the disease but to work with it – to educate myself and understand it. I viewed it not as an enemy but as a process that would surely unfold. The lexicon of war would do me no good. I also didn't allow it to define me. My approach enabled me to recover, and while the illness became chronic and felt interminable, my damaged central nervous system used all of its energy to heal.

There were ups and downs in the treatment process. Infused with aggressive medicine, I spent hours and days partially absent from my own life, conceding precious mothering and writing energy to fever dreams; my life was a procession of days that flowed like Rudyard Kipling's 'great, grey-green, greasy Limpopo River, all set about with fever trees.' In a medicated half-state that was neither here nor there, I hallucinated, and heard voices. One afternoon, a soft animal voice spoke in my ear. 'I comin' down to touches you awake.' The unearthly voice woke me up, but I was not puzzled or afraid. I was being cared for, kept vigil for. That moment, that vision and visitation, was the turning point of my illness.

There were periods of remission, and in 2004 I was strong enough to fulfil a different long-held wish: to become a yoga teacher. I wanted to study with a certain Indian yoga master of a respected lineage, who had an ashram in the US. By chance – by some wild chance – he chose to take his teachings on the road. I studied with him and his daughter at a Zen Buddhist temple in Rhode Island, where I could stay close to my sons. My yoga and meditation practice became an organising principle, strengthening and supporting me as I recovered from a complex illness and its psychological fallout.

Today my body holds just a few reminders: an acute sensitivity to sound, to sudden loud noises and voices, and severe osteoporosis, worsened by a particular and necessary medication. My once robust skeleton resembles a sea creature, a fragile conundrum of hollow coral fingers. One day it might break. But not today.

Recuperation was a long haul, and lonely. I no longer had the teaching community in my life for friendship or support. I had new friends, but found myself longing for the women I had known in Tortola. I left behind a warm island community, where I had come of age as a woman, nurtured by rich, lasting friendships with women I was sharing journeys with – including the momentous journey of becoming mothers together. I became restless, looking for something I couldn't define. I was restive, pawing the ground and sniffing the air, looking this way and that, waiting for life to properly begin again.

I've lived in New England for three decades now, in this quaint, picturesque little city-by-the-sea. I have a wild ocean beach to walk on, where I feel hardy and whole. I've raised two sons, taught in their schools, volunteered with civic and charity organisations. I've written for local, regional and national publications, given readings of my poetry and made presentations from my travels. I've become a US citizen along the way. I've gained rich friendships. But not until five years ago did I begin to send out roots into the Native American soil that has embraced me – no longer piggybacking on the roots that are my sons' genuine legacy. They were both born to this island, while I am an immigrant. It can take a long time to belong, to say the word *home*.

Four years ago, after my second Labrador retriever died, a black Labrador puppy caught my heart off-guard and blew it wide open. I saw the rescue agency photograph and my head spun, and I had to have him in my world. I adopted him the following day, naming him Sachem, a title held by Algonquian and Narragansett tribal chiefs of the North Atlantic coast. The name is also interpreted as *wise leader*. Sachem is my constant, trusty companion. A few years ago, I began to crave the company of horses, too. I rode a little as a child and as a girl, then whenever I could – taking lessons, making room for horse treks when I travelled. On one of our early family visits to Nepal, to a mystical, secluded Tharu village in Chitwan, in the southern lowland territory, we hacked out. It was my first time in the saddle for many years. My sons and my husband were on horseback beside me, or in front or behind – I barely remember, because with every step the horse brought me closer to my original being. The stable hands held my sons' horses on lead ropes and I was able, perhaps for the first time as a mother, to be *off watch*. I was free to enter a state of flow, to be utterly absorbed. I experienced rapture. I was a girl-child again.

Of course, it wasn't wise to ride, given the condition of my bones, but my spirit needed something that horses could offer. I made friends at a nearby stable (in the US they are called barns). I watched lessons and helped with chores, with turnout and feeding. I took lessons and loved it. I was invited to ride out on the ocean beach, and as we trotted on the sand I melted into the horse, like butter. I learned to ride again, learned to canter and soar. A new horse arrived at the barn – a spirited, glorious blue roan appaloosa with a fiery mohawk mane that, to this day, will not lie flat to her shoulder. We blew each other's hearts open. Her name is Sugar. I never found it necessary to change her name. This mare walked into my life to help me send out more tender roots, to help me belong. We talk to each other and I tell her how hard it is sometimes, to be a human. She tells me what it's like to be a horse, and to be a horse around humans.

I committed myself wholeheartedly to my horse, to what was in front of me instead of what was behind me. I came face to face with where I was, with what had been and what no longer *was* in my life – and with what was necessary. And what was necessary was mucking out a horse stall, in humid hot summer and biting cold winter, shovelling manure, getting my hands dirty. I embraced all the elements of New England life. For the first time after my long illness, I felt grounded. Or – as I prefer to call it – *earthed*. I dug deep, got my hands wholesomely dirty, and felt the earth shifting. With time, I regained my strength and vigour. I decided to learn horses from the ground up and from the outside in, a process that is ongoing.

A few years ago, Sugar and I moved to a new barn at a lovely old horse farm. I found myself spending more and more time at the farm, not just with Sugar. I love every aspect of being with horses, even standing with them in their stall, filling water buckets. One horse in particular caught my attention. He was in the stall next to Sugar, and was on indefinite stall rest. Moon was an old horse, doted on by his owner, suffering with a condition that affects the bones of the hoof. He was heavily medicated and failing. I spent time with him, tending to him when his owner could not, and I began to sense his inner energetic state. I watched, saddened, as his interest in life seeped away. One day, I read – intuited – information, written as if on a floating index card held to the inside of my brain, above my eyes. The message referred to Moon's liver, and to an excess of water. I shared this with my friend, the farm manager, who, luckily for me, was receptive. She said that Moon's liver was indeed failing, due to the heavy toll of his medications. As we talked, she reached down to loosen his bandage, and we found his entire foot engorged with fluid. Shortly afterwards, I dreamt that Moon drowned in his stall. The following day he had to be put down.

That was the beginning of my communication with horses. Owners began to ask me to 'read' their horses. I simply get quiet and 'be' with the horse. I see things written on those curious floating index cards; I read words and veterinary terms I have never heard of, and have to research and verify. I pass the information to the experts. I listen to the horses and hear their stories. I sense when they are depressed or overworked, where they hold an invisible, deep-tissue bruise or a looming colic – which I sometimes experience as pain in my own gut. I run my hands above their spine and my hands tingle and burn, telling me where energy is pulsing or stuck. I hold their head in a certain way that I was never taught, cup their eyes in my palm, and the horse drops its head and falls asleep on my arm. It is energy healing, simply. It is exciting, rewarding and curiously unsurprising, just a wholly natural process. I experience a similar communication with dogs – whether known to me or new – who run to me and greet me like an old friend.

It has been a rich discovery, to know that I can use my intuitive energy in this way. After a lifetime of being fey, subduing and hiding and even fearing my psychic energy, I feel whole and authentic. I am not an interloper in the world but part of it – part of its ecosystem and part of its whole. The farm, with its sturdy stone barns, built around 1900, is in a rural part of Aquidneck Island that reminds me a lot of Yorkshire. I feel at home there. And there, with the horses, my Tourette tics disappear. They simply melt away.

Some years ago I casually picked up a book about synaesthesia, a benign neurological condition in which, to put it simply, when one sense is activated, another unrelated sense is activated at the same time. This may, for example, take the form of hearing music and simultaneously sensing the sound as swirls or patterns of colour. It is estimated that four percent of humans have some form of synaesthesia, most commonly grapheme-colour synesthaesia, in which letters and numbers are associated with specific colours or patterns. Discovering this was a revelation, and I immediately associated it with Tourette Syndrome as a privilege of neurodivergence: I had assumed, all my life, that everyone saw and experienced numerical digits and letters of the alphabet in consistent colour, and that it was perfectly normal for the name of each weekday to be associated with a unique colour, shape and texture.

I then learned about mirror-touch synaesthesia, which has been described as a kind of supercharged empathy: a person feels as though they're being touched if they witness it happening to someone else. It can be benign – an observed advantage in recognising facial expressions, for example – or burdensome, as in the case of a neurologist who felt intense pressure in his chest when he saw a patient receiving CPR.

My synaesthesia informs my experience of communicating and receiving information from horses, and feeling their discomfort as a bodily or emotional experience. I also experience deep pressure in my chest and abdomen as I watch ocean tides encroaching, receding and reversing. I have consulted neurologists about my 'discovery' and experience and their counsel has always been simple: enjoy this gift and privilege. For the first time in my life, I feel that I can.

Last summer, my husband and I walked on the trails at Sachuest Point, a wildlife refuge above my ocean beach. The air was clear and the views were stunning. 'Let's sit on the grass and watch the ocean,' I said. 'But we wouldn't want to disturb the ecosystem,' replied my husband. I was indignant. 'I'm a paid-up, card-carrying member of the ecosystem!' I have come to feel that I am *of* this New England land, of this ancient First Nation territory. I love it and care passionately for it. It holds a profound energy. I talk to its trees and to the horses, and to Sachem, my dog, and we are a tribe. We are not wild – we are untamed together. Our spirits are free. This island is home to my sons and now to me. I belong. Here I am by the wild ocean, with the trees and the grass, and the dogs and horses, and even the ants. We keep vigil, together. And I say for the first time, 'I Am!'

As I finish writing this story, I am unpacking my bags after a two-week visit to Nepal. With my husband and our sons and our older son's fiancée, and my husband's siblings and their children, I walked to Thyangboche, the exquisite Tibetan Buddhist monastery that sits on a hillside in the Everest region, at 12,670 feet. We trekked for five days, climbing more than three thousand feet through villages and rhododendron forests, on paths of leaves and up countless stone steps that were set into the hillside by human hands. We carried my mother-in-law's ashes because it was her wish to go to rest on that serene hillside where she, too, walked, many years ago. The pilgrimage was joyous, if physically challenging, and the air was as clean as any I have tasted. The mountain paths are steep, up and down, and one day our sirdar *chose a shortcut and we ran out of path. We scrambled up the hillside, grasping boulders and scrub on the way. It was everything that I once could not even have dreamt of asking my body to do. It was gruelling, and glorious. My legs and my lungs met the challenge, and my spirits soared as I climbed the last few steps to the monastery.*

The following morning we were allowed to attend the puja ceremony for the recently deceased Rinpoche of the monastery. The ceremony was long and loud and profoundly intimate, and moved me to tears and other, new emotions. I was mesmerised by the sound of the monks, chanting, their deep voices emanating from the core of the earth, punctuated by the blowing of horns and clanging of cymbals. I willingly drowned in the reverberations. I was bathed in ritual sound and in the energy of pure intention. Afterwards, I felt that I had been explored and discovered by a marvellous journey, like a newly forged path, or a smooth marble sculpture from which everything that was not me had been chiselled away and cast to the winds. I emerged into the sunlight clear-headed and brave, with a fierce awareness of my life force, wondering where in the world this strong body and untamed spirit will take me next.

14

JANE'S STORY:
MRS K EATS HER WAY
AROUND ITALY

*The menopause comes… But then you're free, no longer a slave, no
longer a machine with parts. You're just a person, in business… It is
horrendous, but then it's magnificent.*

Phoebe Waller-Bridge, *Fleabag*, spoken by Belinda Frears

Jane responded to my call for entries in the Bradt e-zine in 2021.
Initially we were unable to meet due to Covid restrictions and
then because, well, we were both off travelling! We shared some
wonderful, raucous Zoom sessions discussing the bumpy road
through menopause and our shared pleasure at shifting from being
good, dutiful mothers and grandmothers to becoming women in our
own right, seizing every opportunity that comes our way. We both
expressed how we feel more ourselves than ever before. I admire
Jane's tenacity, too. I really hope we can meet in person before
too long.

It's a delicious irony that Jane's (aka Mrs K) adventures as a
travel writer should start with *Woman and Home*. The magazine was
running a competition – and Jane knew exactly why she wanted to
be the one to win the prize.

One thing I have learned first-hand is that menopause does not run to any kind of schedule. I began to *feel* different in my late thirties and early forties but my periods didn't stop until I was fifty-seven and I didn't start getting any serious menopausal symptoms until I was sixty. Doctors scratch their heads and frown at me, but I've heard other women with similar stories. It's important for women to know that menopause is fickle and idiosyncratic and that it can last for many, many years. When my children became a little more independent, I started to feel restless. I began to feel that I could have done better for myself – that I wanted to prove myself, that there was something else 'out there'. Perhaps I was in perimenopause – it certainly felt as if I was on the cusp of change.

One day I simply announced that I'd applied to do a BA in Humanities with The Open University (OU). Everyone except my mother was surprised. She always believed in me, even when I didn't. When I was young, she used to tell me, 'You'd make a good journalist.' I think she recognised that I was beginning to grow into myself.

My life followed a pattern like millions of other women. I was a bright girl, but I didn't do as well academically as I could have done. I always knew the answers in school, but I didn't like putting my hand up. I married at twenty-one and started a family at twenty-five. My parents encouraged me at school, but I was more interested in boys and having fun. I went to the local college and then worked in the DHSS office – it was boring, routine stuff. Then I went into retail, which I quite enjoyed because I love talking to people, but the hours were long and inflexible. When I started to work at the local Waterstones bookshop, I felt more at home. I'd always loved English and history and was an avid reader, so it suited me well.

I managed to pay for the OU degree from my wages. It wasn't as expensive then as it is now. This started a very hectic, exciting six years of my life. I can't imagine now how I found time to go to work every day, look after the children, and get all the course work done – but I did. I absolutely loved studying. The foundation year was an introduction to the arts: English, History, Music, etc. Gradually I was drawn to History of Art. I'm not artistically creative but I was captivated by the lives of artists.

I started visiting galleries in London. Looking at art challenged my thinking and gave me permission to explore the big themes in my life. I looked at the work of Artemisia Gentileschi, a seventeenth-century Italian painter who suffered rape, torture and public humiliation and yet continued to defy the establishment in Rome to make her voice heard. Perhaps she used her art to seek revenge and to show themes that previously had only been painted by men for the male gaze. She painted strong women who challenged societal norms. They were survivors rising above the most terrifying experiences. It seemed to me that if women like Artemisia Gentileschi could rise, then so could I.

The first OU summer school I attended was a revelation. It was the first time I'd been away from home just as myself, with no children or husband to look after. I was not a mum or a wife while I was there – I had no caring responsibilities. I was a fully grown-up independent adult for that one week. It may have been only one week, but in terms of its significance it was huge. Summer school took place at Royal Holloway College; it was like a chateau, complete with a gallery displaying Pre-Raphaelite paintings, which we were studying that year. It was perfect, and utterly wonderful to just be me, losing myself in learning and following my passions.

I was drawn more and more to Italian Renaissance art, and that's what I focused on in my final year.

After six years of part-time study, in my mid-forties, I graduated. The ceremony was elating. Baroness Betty Boothroyd, Chancellor of The Open University at that time, conferred my degree; I could hardly believe that I'd done it. I was so proud, and I didn't want to take off the graduation gown. I wanted that moment to last for as long as possible – it gave me such a sense of status.

After graduating I felt a bit lost. I missed the course and my fellow students. While they were moving on to careers in teaching and so on, I still wasn't sure of my direction. I still had responsibilities at home but I continued to read about Italy and Renaissance art. I travelled to Italy as often as my annual leave would allow. It was important to me not to lose momentum and so I decided to return to the OU to do a one-year Italian language course.

I was casually leafing through a copy of *Woman and Home* magazine one day and my attention was grabbed by a competition they were running: 'Dare to be Different'. *If you could do anything you wanted, what would it be?* I knew exactly what I wanted. I sat on my bed with a notepad and pen and wrote my submission from the heart. All my feelings about longing to study in Florence flowed out. I wrote about how I'd fallen in love with Renaissance Art. I explained that I was yearning to learn more by studying at the British Institute of Florence – that was the thing I really wanted to do, but I had children and couldn't afford to do it. I never thought for one moment that I would win, but I thought it was worth a try.

My husband came to pick me up from work one day and told me that he'd had a phone call from a magazine to say we'd won a holiday in Italy. There wasn't a gentle way to correct him with, 'I've won a study-trip to Florence!' The prize included a British Airways business class flight and two weeks of study at the British Institute of Florence. I still remember how I felt on the plane – I think I knew it was the beginning of something momentous for me. It seemed unbelievable and I was on cloud nine. I was also aware that with all that free alcohol the hostess was offering, I didn't want to create a bad impression with the representative from the British Institute who was meeting me! (I wasn't so restrained on the flight home.) I gasped as we approached Florence and I caught my first glimpse of the Duomo. I was here, in this city I had dreamt of for so long. This was me, I had taken a risk, entered a competition, declared what I wanted to do – and I had arrived.

Being in Florence on my own was initially quite scary. It was before I had a mobile phone and so I was cut off from my family. This was a new me, one I was learning to embrace. I was a solo traveller. I immersed myself in all things Florence, walking for miles around the city and visiting all the galleries. I didn't have much money to live on, so I had to be careful about expenditure. With less food and huge amounts of walking, I went home half a stone lighter! I made a friend – Helen – while I was there, and twenty years later we still meet up in London each year. We usually visit art galleries together, but one time we also spent a few hours in Highgate cemetery, soaking up the wild garlic and the Gothic tombstones. I'm not sure what we were thinking that day!

My time in Florence was the start of my metamorphosis. I wouldn't have missed it for the world. The course at the British Institute of Florence involved a mixture of Italian language lessons, lectures and visits to galleries with expert guides. It brought all my academic study to life: here I was, seeing all this sublime art in the flesh. This was my wonderland, where all my years of study came alive. It was also the place where a few crystals started to form in my thinking.

Enough seeds were sown while I was in Florence for me to start seeing myself differently, to wonder, perhaps, if I could create a new path for myself. I bought every book and video I could afford about Italy and took several short courses on travel writing. I met many people from different backgrounds who previously I might have found intimidating, but I was beginning to feel a bit more secure and confident in my own right. I was starting to feel that I had something to contribute.

I travelled to Italy as often as I could with my husband, but it wasn't until seven or eight years after my degree, when the children had left home and life had become a bit easier, that I turned my attention to wondering if *I* could be a travel writer. I got the chance to reduce my working hours and decided that this was my opportunity: with part-time work, I thought, I could really give travel writing a go. I used to tell my bookshop colleagues that my dream job would be to go to Italy and get paid for it – and now I am! It's still hard to take that in.

I started to hear a little voice in my head, an inner champion telling me that I had nothing to lose. Writing is not like starting a business – there's no associated financial risk. I listed my strengths: I knew a lot about Italy, I owned a small library of books, and we had a computer and internet access at home. Most importantly I have a passion for Italy, and as an older woman I have a lot of life experience that informs my writing and can give it a fresh angle. It's more real – I put my heart and soul into it. I decided it was now or never and it was well worth a try!

So, shortly before we set off on a holiday to Sicily, I took the plunge and sent a pitch to *Italia* magazine. I'd made a connection with the editor, and we'd had some friendly email exchanges. I was thrilled when she accepted my pitch: 'Six days in Sicily'. We went to the west coast, to Trapani, Erice and Marsala. Without really knowing it, I had jumped in at the deep end – the Mafia presence was still strong, although you could feel that the Sicilians were pushing back. There was a lot to navigate. The area is also known for its cuisine. Erice, for example, is famous for its marzipan fruits. Mafia and food – a baptism of fire for me as a writer! This was my idea of heaven and I think I began to adopt my 'Mrs K eats her way around Italy' identity there and then. Who wouldn't choose to eat their way around Italy?

At the age of fifty-four I saw my first article printed in *Italia*, set with lots of glossy pictures. I was so proud, a little shocked even – I bought six copies! Once you have one article in print it gives you credibility as a writer. I probably bored people to tears about it, but it was so big for me. It amuses me now that I'm quite blasé when I see one of my articles in print, though I still tend to buy one copy of the publication – it still gives me pride to see it on the shelf. In the early days of my writing my mum would proofread my copy for me, until I grew more confident. She made suggestions and cheered me on. That made a big difference – I think we all need a mum or a friend or confidante to cheer us on – as raising a family can really sap your confidence about becoming an independent woman in the world. We get so used to our identity being bound up with a role we sometimes forget that we are individuals too.

Another important element in my personal growth also happened in my early fifties. I badly needed to get fit and to do that I needed an incentive and a goal. So, I signed up to climb three volcanoes for charity: Mount Etna, Vesuvius and Stromboli. I was the girl who 'skived off' sport at school – I am very unfit – so it was a real challenge for me. The local gym gave me free membership in exchange for publicity, so I wrote regular updates about my progress in the local press – reports on my goals, on my fitness levels and how much weight I'd lost. It was the incentive I needed to set my targets and make myself accountable – scary and exposing, but it worked. After a year of training, aged fifty-three, I was climbing those volcanoes! Very often on the way up I thought that I'd never make it, but I did. I huffed and puffed my way up and my sense of achievement was huge. I'd met my goals and changed the way I thought about myself. I encountered some interesting people, mostly much younger and fitter than me, but nonetheless I achieved what they did. I was starting to own myself, to be less shy. I had to share cabins with strangers and learn to be comfortable and honest about who I am.

I continued to study, taking short courses that introduced me to the mechanics of how to get travel writing published; what editors want to see in a pitch and how to demonstrate to them that I should be the person to write it. We were shown the pitfalls to avoid, how many ideas to send, and so on. There was so much to learn. I had never heard of 'FAM' or 'familiarisation' trips – free trips provided to the media by travel operators and tourist boards to showcase the best they have to offer – but I soon learned how enriching they can be.

I'd read a novel set by Lake Orta, northwest of Milan. Lake Orta is less well known than lakes Garda and Como, so I hoped that might help me 'pitch it'. I decided to organise a press trip for myself. I wrote to all the local tourist boards, and they set me up with hotels and trips to see the area. Subsequently, I've been on other kinds of press trips where groups of journalists are taken to a resort or a specific area. They tend to be really hectic because the company behind the trip is trying to get its money's worth – and they also tend to be full of boozy journalists, who are quite hard to keep up with! On other trips you're invited to go on a vacation, just like any other guest. My first one of those was to Assisi. It was wonderful – like a holiday, and with plenty of time to explore and write.

As soon I set off on a work trip and I'm on the plane, the sense of freedom is joyous. In fact, the moment I get on the train to Stansted Airport my energy levels start to rise. My favourite press trip was to Siena before the Palio. I wrote an article for the *Daily Mail* taking the angle that the build-up to the race, with all its traditions, was an event in itself. Work trips are intense: there's a pressure not only to get engaging photos, to complete accurate research, but also to capture the 'feel' and 'smell' of the place with local colour and undiscovered gems. I take a lot of notes and produce many drafts before I am happy. Other than that it really is like a vacation!

I pitched *Italia* magazine to write about the witch trials in the Italian Alps near Liguria. The witch trials in the municipality of Triora between 1587 and 1589 were some of the bloodiest in the Liguria region. In 1587 Triora was gripped by famine and poverty. A group of women – medicine women, herbalists and wise women – lived together in seclusion in the poorest part of the city. The women were accused of having relations with the devil, causing pestilence and acid rain, even being cannibals. Four of them were executed and some died in prison. This was an important article for me to write, bringing home to me that some attitudes to older women still haven't really changed.

My shy twenty-year-old self would not have believed that I would be doing this in my mid-sixties. But my younger self wasn't ready. She needed time, experience and confidence – and probably lower levels of oestrogen – to become 'selfish' enough to do it. I read an article that suggested that lower levels of oestrogen and progesterone post menopause make us less inclined to nurturing and homemaking, that we feel less drawn to the domestic and more attracted to the world outside the home. That certainly rings true for me. I no longer feel that I was the one who didn't achieve anything and ended up in mundane jobs. Now, with my lower levels of oestrogen, I feel angry about the scandalous way women are treated, not least we 'WASPI' women – Women against State Pension Inequality – who, born in the 1950s, were not given sufficient warning in order to protect our retirements in the light of dramatic changes in the state pension age.

I think my late flourishing came as quite a shock to my husband, but he has been supportive. He's grown used to me flying off on press trips and him being the one left behind. But he also loves it when we can go together – he enjoys a holiday while I'm at work making notes, taking photos and looking for interesting angles. My husband does his share of looking after the grandchildren. I'm still a nurturing mother and a loving grandmother but I'm not pulled in the same way as I once was. This is my time now.

My post-menopausal career has changed me. Sometimes I feel like Cinderella; there I am strutting around Italy on press trips, staying in posh hotels with well-known journalists – and then I come home to cleaning the toilet and wiping the grandchildren's bottoms. But the older I get the more I don't care anymore! Each year I go to the International Media Marketplace, which is essentially like speed-dating for travel media professionals. As a travel writer you schedule appointments with travel companies and tourist boards from all over the world. At first it felt overwhelming, but now I swan around confidently. I feel like a different person. It's been a gradual flourishing – I've learnt how to be me.

Recently I set up my own business – Boston History Tours. Not many people know Boston in Lincolnshire, and I believe I can use my skills as a travel writer to bring the town to life. It has a rich and fascinating history. We offer guided walking tours for the general public, and I guide several school groups each week. I also run the occasional travel writing workshop. I always tell the participants to just go for it – that they have nothing to lose! Like me, they tend to think you need a degree in journalism or a private school education to be part of that 'set' – but *I'm* not from that background, and *I've* done it.

I work part-time in Fydell House, a beautiful Queen Anne house in the centre of Boston which is where my tours of Boston start. One day I came up with the idea of the Boston Book Festival. Together with some very energetic friends we launched the first festival in September 2021, with Benjamin Zephaniah, Michael Morpurgo and Milly Johnson as our first guest writers. It's been a huge success, and it's another way that I feel I can promote my home town.

The competition title 'Dare to be Different' has come true for me. I am now a travel writer; I am Director of Boston History Tours and I am the instigator and Chairperson of the Boston Book Festival! If you'd told me when I was a young shop assistant in Waterstones that this is what I would be doing at sixty-five, I would not have believed you. Or maybe I would – maybe I just needed to say it out loud and to be heard. I think it's taken a long time to allow myself to hear and inhabit my own dreams.

15

JORJ'S STORY:

HONOURING THE MATRIARCHS

'Cut your cloth and sew it together.'

Julie East John (Jorj's mother)

'Free for the strangest adventures' was, in many ways, Jorj's life-long mantra. When these adventures came to an abrupt end, Jorj was required to see her world from another viewpoint and to forge a different definition of adventure. Her story is a reverse take on the others – she *was* leading the life she loved and had to reframe that by making major life changes in quick succession.

Like all the best narrators, Jorj challenged my perceptions and life view every time we met. As soon as we were at liberty to, we met up for a walk in Mortimer Forest near Ludlow. It turned out to be symbolic – every path we took was either closed to the public or led us back to the car park, before we even had the chance to lose ourselves in our stories of the labyrinths of life. After about six attempts we gave up and had a coffee in my van!

As Jorj recounts the story of her life over the last twenty years, we can see that, while her circumstances have changed, a number of times her spirit of adventure has never dulled – she remains intrepid, facing reality with equanimity, constantly appraising and planning routes in and out of troubled waters. She is still challenging herself, open to new ideas, able to advise and inspire others – all the while holding fast to her ethical precepts.

I was born in Phoenix, Arizona, but I lived in California for most of my childhood and early adulthood. I had a passion for creating things and although I studied design at university, I decided to keep artistic pursuits for pleasure and went on for to study for a degree in finance. Finance is black and white – it was a clearer, calmer early path for me, and it didn't threaten my sense of self as much as criticism of my creativity did. I then went on to have a career in communications and public relations, much of which, of course, needs creative flair.

As life has gone on, I have really valued the skills that both of these disciplines have offered me. I worked for one of San Diego's largest PR companies where I was responsible for a lot of their maritime work, including a contract involving three ferries for use in Hong Kong. When I was asked to relocate to the UK for two years to manage the marketing and contract for this, I jumped at the chance.

I fell in love with the UK the minute I set foot here. I loved its size and the proximity to Europe and the rest of the world. I loved its strong moral values, although I'm not sure those still apply in the same way. Two years extended to four years, as they do, and then I was able to apply for UK residency – my daughter was six when we came here, and I wanted her to be educated in the UK. She was able to have a proper old-school childhood here, to go outside with other kids and play without the pressures that a Californian life brings with it, without having to grow up too quickly. Things have changed since then, but at that time she was able to have an idyllic childhood and a fabulous education.

Setting up my own agency felt like the natural next step. I established my marketing communications consultancy, Rowland Main, using my grandmothers' maiden names. Sadly, neither of them was alive at the time, but I knew that they would have felt proud and honoured. My mother, of course, was very pleased. I know that without these strong women, whose remarkable strength and commitment influenced my development, I wouldn't be where I am today. The older I get, the more I recognise the role that female elders have played in my life.

I'm typical of the Americans who grew up predominantly in the 50s and 60s – there was a big fitness kick back then and that suited me just fine. Always a water baby, as a child I would 'fall in' to every stream, river, pond or puddle I saw. My sport of choice has always been anything to do with water: in it, on it or under it! I started to 'paddle' in my teens – I became a canoeist, a kayaker, and then a whitewater kayaker. I love travel and, eventually, in my forties, earned my qualification as a safety kayaker, becoming part of a very small worldwide expedition community who would head out to specific rivers to assess risk and hazard and gather information. I worked like a Trojan with my PR company for nine months of each year and then took three months out to do my expedition work. My clients knew this was my schedule and together we made it happen. I continued like this into my fifties; many of my military clients were amused to encounter an 'old' woman safety kayaker. Compared with them I *was* old! They had a healthy respect for me and every expedition was amazing in its own right. I adored my work life: both the challenges of being a PR consultant and the passion I felt for safety kayaking.

The fitness requirements for those sorts of trips is really demanding, so I had a personal trainer to get me to the right level.

At one point I was training for an expedition to Borneo when out of the blue we were notified that it had been cancelled due to an insurrection in the remote river valley we had been due to visit. My trainer said, 'Never mind, we're not wasting all this effort – get on this erg (rowing machine) while we have a think.' His thoughts were that I should enter the 2002 C.R.A.S.H.-B. Sprints World Indoor Rowing Championships. *My* thoughts were, 'Yeah, right. I'm going to sit on this stupid machine that goes absolutely nowhere and is the hardest anaerobic exercise there is – are you out of your mind?' He said, 'Yep, just do it' – and I did! At the age of fifty-three I did as I was told and competed in both the UK and the world championships. I won a bronze medal in both, which was kind of bizarre! It still didn't endear me to machine rowing, though, so when I came back and 'hung up' my erg, to maintain my fitness, I started running. That set my dominoes tumbling. I should have stuck to rowing!

I developed problems with my feet, which was frustrating and went on for about seven years before I got a diagnosis. It was a simple condition requiring an operation on both feet, which was successful. Unfortunately, my stitches got infected and I got MRSA and then sepsis. It was devastating. I couldn't walk and then needed more surgery – I was virtually immobile for two years and lost all the muscle conditioning I had gained. In this period I lived on a smallholding – it was my life's dream to live this way and a terrible bereavement not to be able to look after the land. I was even having to go up and down the stairs on my bottom. I realised that if I couldn't get my fitness back, I would have to give this place up, which was a heartbreaking thought.

My upbringing stood me in good stead at this point. We were taught never to impose limitations on what we could do. The central tenet of my upbringing was accountability – whatever I did, good, bad or indifferent, I had to be accountable. And that accountability is what keeps the balance. I believe it's all down to me. Some might call this being a control freak. I see it as having ownership of myself! So, I started a full-fledged campaign to get my fitness back. I was sixty-six and it took eighteen months of working so damn hard. But I did it – I got it back. I worked every day on improving my core strength, my balance, muscle tone and flexibility. It wasn't initially about being gym-fit; it was about being functionally fit – to once again be able to manage the day-to-day things that I needed to do to successfully run a smallholding single-handed.

My mother and her mother and my paternal grandmother were all strong, take-charge, no-nonsense women. Most of my family-line is European in origin but I know I also have Native American genes. Having that bloodline has always been a source of pride for me – I don't know why, because it's nothing that I did! I knew of my Cherokee connection from about the age of ten and when I had a choice of subject matter for school projects, I would often choose one with an indigenous Indian connection – bushcraft, natural science, food and culture. Cherokee society is matrilineal; children take the clan of their mother. Women are the property owners in the family and the men join them in their mother's household. Mothers, not fathers, have control over children and property. This made perfect sense to me. My immediate family of origin was traditionally patriarchal; however, I believe these distant roots run deep. When I was in my mid-teens a family member researched our ancestry and discovered a Pocahontas link, and it became a great sense of pride that I knew my background going back thirteen generations

– conveniently ignoring the less salubrious bits that also appeared along the way!

Despite my city upbringing, I have always had a very keen affinity with the natural world and have tried as hard as I can to work in harmony with nature. Being connected to the earth, her seas and soil, is essential to me. I love sitting absolutely stock still in the countryside for ages and ages. I know people complain about feeling invisible as they get older, but it does have its advantages – being able to observe the natural world without being disturbed is a deep pleasure. I have learned over the years how to forage safely – despite one mushroom incident I would rather forget – and create tasty stuff virtually from nothing! I would love to think my proclivities are genetic, but I also know when you are really interested in something it is easy to absorb learning.

I've always valued women in my life. My mother was such a strong influence. She's the one that formed me, and she was formed by her mother. One of her early achievements was to co-found a bank start-up, technically a 'Savings and Loan', in California. The whole board was made up of women – I never thought about that before linking all this together. So, I suppose I grew up absorbing all this, like a sponge. She was determined, successful, brave – a woman in her own right, which gave me permission to be the same.

After getting my fitness back I started to reflect on what I had gained from rehabilitating myself. I knew that I had succeeded not because I was special or different, but because I was determined and committed to hold on to my dream. I had been totally bloody-minded in taking control of my thoughts and what was going on in my head. My mental default position when I started was 'I can't, I can't!' It took a while and lots of effort, but finally I retrained my brain's refrain to become 'How can I? *How* can I?' – and then '*This* is how!' It took time, patience and stubbornness, but ultimately I found ways that got me where I needed to be. Now I could start living again. It was time to try a new venture.

I realised that I had learned a valuable lesson. I might be older, but I had brought myself back from a completely disabling condition. I had come to understand the importance of functional fitness – which I had never given a thought to before – and I now wanted to share with others how to do more easily the everyday tasks that depend on balance, core strength, mobility and flexibility. Those skills are all so essential to maintaining quality of life, whatever challenges someone might be facing. I decided that I had something worth sharing with other people who might have given up on themselves.

Before advising anyone else I knew the only way to become credible was to get qualified. I signed up for every qualification I needed – I concurrently studied anatomy, physiology, nutrition, the needs of older adults and exercise referrals for various conditions (stroke, heart attack, COPD, diabetes, obesity and many others). In my cohort of students, the next oldest in the group to me was forty-two and she saw herself as old! I was cramming as fast as I could – holy moly, the flashcards came out until I knew my stuff inside out and passed the exams.

Helping people regain mobility and improve functional fitness is different from teaching gym fitness. To me there is no difference between teaching functional fitness and safety kayaking – you have people's lives in your hands and it's a big responsibility. I knew my heart was with the over-sixties – they are the ones who have been sold a bill of goods. The messaging out there is you're old, so you should expect to lose muscle mass, fitness, flexibility. It's bollocks.

Don't you dare tell me you can't – you can, you just might have to do it another way. It's true our physiology changes as we age – rest and nutrition become even more important for progression and recovery, for example. Even so, it's crucial to think not 'I can't', but instead, '*How can I?*'.

By May 2019 I was fully qualified, and so I set up AAA (Active Ageing Agency), using my savings to fund the start-up stage of my business plan. I quickly gained contracts with care homes where I was to design individual fitness plans for the residents. I was presented with so many different conditions that I was able to build my experience and skill quickly. Finding the appropriate kind of movement and activities to help clients live their lives more enjoyably, comfortably, happily, safely and with more confidence was so rewarding! Both the carers and I were amazed at how quickly the work made a difference, especially to the residents with dementia – it improved their sense of well-being and their memory function and reduced their agitation and outbursts.

I had one stroke client who as a younger man had played county water polo. When we swam together, at first he walked his laps insisting that he couldn't swim. It was a case of him persuading his brain to 'walk his legs' while horizontal in the water – essentially doing the flutter kick – and then persuading his arms to come over his head too. He just needed to access a different part of his brain. For motivation I challenged him to beat me in a race – a month later, he wiped the floor with me! I have never been so happy to lose. One other chap with advanced dementia didn't engage with anyone or anything. One day I was working with other clients in the room, and I caught a flicker in his eye – I had a boxing glove on. Unknown to any of us, he had been a boxer; a memory was stirred in him and we started to spar with each other. One day, out of the blue, he started really punching out and I had to brace myself. It was the first time he had made eye contact with anyone, and he had a huge smile on his face. After the session and out of sight, the carers and I all cried – in that moment he had been able to relive his boxing career.

One woman with dementia and very little coordination observed me playing catch with another of my clients. I could tell she was interested, so I asked her if she would like a go – and she caught the ball. I thought that was amazing. As she tried to throw it back she looked very confused. I took her hand, the one that was holding the ball, and led it back and forth a couple times to try and find the memory of that motion in her brain. The concentration on that woman's face while she held that ball and squeezed it, muttering, 'Throw, throw'… I was standing quite close, so wherever it went would be fine. What I never dreamt is that her right leg would kick out – and I ended up with a bruise that almost flattened me. I couldn't cry out or fall because that would really upset her. When she looked down at her hands she saw she was still holding the ball. Even though she was saying 'throw', what her brain heard was 'kick'!

Every visit and every client were very different. Some days they wouldn't want to talk at all but, if I quietly observed their behaviour in that moment, I could usually pick up on how they were feeling. They might be mithering or just gently rubbing their hands and I could then work out then what movement might make an improvement. Sometimes they would be absolutely transfixed with something visual, like a specific colour, or something tactile like a scarf to get their fingers moving.

They were more receptive to me that I had any right to expect. And that's because I made no demands, had no expectations. Rarely did they remember my name despite seeing me the day before – mostly they didn't remember their own name – but that's irrelevant. All I was there for was to try and give them more functional movement.

Soon I had more than enough work for one person. All the care homes were giving me great feedback, telling me I was providing exactly what their clients needed. Many of the staff were interested themselves in the kind of training I was offering, and for me that is key – having qualified trainers who know that the first challenge is to understand people's mental state and then become deeply invested in improving their functional fitness. Active Ageing Agency took off rapidly. It was in big demand, and I was at the point of expanding – training and taking on new staff. I felt validated and excited.

Then, in the spring of 2020, on top of the Covid pandemic, which immediately closed care homes, my life was further upended. I was branded by the government for being over seventy and was stamped as 'vulnerable'. It was an intolerable situation for me, taking away all my purpose in one mandatory swipe. I had studied and trained for the last few years to set up my business, and now I found myself within just a few months of launching it having to close it down again. Never in my whole life have I let my age define me – my response to any ageist remark has always been *ppwwh* – and now it was imposed upon me. That unjustified 'vulnerable' brand came with obligatory, insurmountable insurance limitations which not only decimated AAA but made me unemployable as well.

There was huge demand for my new business and my original plan was after three years to attempt to sell it to one of the big healthcare providers. I understand that these were exceptional times, that the risks were real and deadly. But there I was, left without work or money and living alone. My purpose had been torn away. My new business, which had grown exponentially faster than my business plan predicted, had to be suspended overnight.

After the first lockdown, when restrictions eased, I tried to get an ordinary job, but because of my 'vulnerable' status I couldn't. I had savings which I'd earmarked for building my business, but during the two years of pandemic I had to live off them. I have a very small pension and therefore I had to supplement my rent from my savings. I knew I had to downsize and find something cheaper, but it was proving impossible. Country properties in lockdown became boltholes for city dwellers, who priced me out. I'm quite reclusive, someone who needs total privacy. I enjoy meeting and working with people, but I can only do that if for the rest of the time I am on my own. At the point when I was within £2.60 and twenty-four hours of being homeless, I began to feel that my quality of life was not acceptable and that it was time to draw it to a close. Although the pandemic was easing, it would be a while before care homes could allow non-essential strangers in and there weren't enough hours in the day to train enough private one-to-one clients to make a living.

At that point serendipity walked in the door. A local farmer offered to put a roof over my head and that gave me a huge reason to be thankful. And then Tash Acres, a graphic designer I'd known since my marketing days, got in touch to ask for my help. Tash wanted to enter a competition run by the Brooks running shoes brand. They were asking for ideas dreamt up while out on a run: an idea that would change 'a life, a day or the world'.

An enthusiastic runner, Tash was bothered by the fact that most races give out badly fitting T-shirts and medals that tend to end up in landfill. She wanted to submit a proposition to change the way we think about running and the exercise we already do. Her plan was to set up a social enterprise and she wanted help with fundraising, marketing, PR and a business perspective, which of course has been my area of expertise for many years. I was able to help Tash shape her idea and give her the confidence that it could become a real thing. And most importantly to remind her that unless she entered she couldn't win!

The idea obviously caught the judges' attention and it won the Brooks competition: Earth Runs was born! It's a really simple concept: to motivate runners, walkers or rollers not with giveaways of useless 'stuff' but by marking their achievements by planting trees where they are most needed across the globe. Every race or challenge a person undertakes earns them trees to be planted, thus harnessing the power of thousands of runners' miles to help fight climate change and support the communities who do the planting. Each runner has an account where they can see the impact they've made with their miles and how many trees they've planted. The programme also includes outreach in schools, encouraging the students to get fitter and improve their mental health while also planting trees and learning about the impact of their efforts. For those that do like a keepsake, there is an Earth Runs biodegradable medal impregnated with British wildflower seeds which can be planted in order to grow flowers for the bees. Even the ribbon is biodegradable. It's both a lovely metaphor and can literally help the environment rather than become part of the problem. I am now largely running the medal side of the business, which is booming – or perhaps I should say blossoming... I am rushed off my feet with it and I haven't even launched our marketing initiatives yet!

At seventy-three, out of nowhere and almost overnight, I am at the heart of a new business that chimes completely with my love of nature and fitness. I feel that I am doing my small bit towards healing this planet by planting trees and reducing waste. It feeds my sense of responsibility and accountability for myself and the earth.

As a child, learning to sew at my mother's knee, I was impatient and impetuous. She kept me on track by unpicking my mistakes (chopping off bits of fabric if they didn't line up, for example!), explaining where I had gone wrong and catching me back up to where I had got to. It's taken me a while and is still a work in progress, but I like to hope I've learned from those days – I have to cut my cloth and sew it together accordingly. It's a great feeling.

16

LESLEY'S STORY:
A HEART-LED LIFE

One's life has value so long as one attributes value to the life of others,
by means of love, friendship, indignation, compassion.

Simone de Beauvoir, *The Coming of Age*

There's nowhere more energising or bracing than Cape Cornwall on a wild spring day. After the long endurance of the Covid lockdown Lesley and I welcomed the simple pleasure of walking and talking. We were meeting so that I could hear more of Lesley's story of how she started her second spring in a new location, with a new career and fresh philosophy of life. Our walk together was also part of my own journey in self-understanding – I had started to think about writing my own eulogy, to give myself perspective, possibly not a wise thing to do on a very blustery day high up on the South West Coast Path. After a few hours of exhilarating cliff walking, we headed back to St Just. Neither the cold nor the wind prevented us from enjoying a Moomaid of Zennor ice cream on a bench outside a small café. Like the path we had just taken, Lesley's story touched me with its precarious nature, its ups and downs, but mostly with the wonderful perspective she got from the top. The sugar hit of the ice cream ended our conversation on a high: burlesque, sex in the lives of crones, and riotous living. A life fully lived.

I was born with a hole in my heart. That meant I wasn't supposed to run, play or do anything energetic, though as I had six siblings the house was never quiet. I was raised in a blended family of seven children. My mum and dad each brought two children into this new family, then together they had me and my two younger sisters. Life was very happy, if a bit chaotic, within the limits of our council house. We lived in a small village close to Manchester airport, and until just a few years ago my whole life was lived in the Manchester area. We lived in an affluent area but we weren't well-off at all. I didn't notice this until I started school and met other children – then some differences became apparent.

I didn't have a lot of energy as a child and I missed lots of school because of hospital appointments and stays. I was ten years old before I could have an operation, and in those days teachers didn't send work home. I didn't like primary school. I needed extra reading and spelling lessons, which made me feel different. My experience of secondary school was similar – I was always on the back foot, having to catch up. I don't think I was a born academic and I didn't excel at a particular subject, though I definitely leaned towards words and not figures.

After leaving school I went to secretarial college and then joined the shorthand-typing pool of a very traditional textile company with a lot of other girls and a 'clocking-off' bell. I worked my way up to supporting management teams and then worked as an executive personal assistant right up until the time when I felt I wanted to change direction.

I met my husband when I was fifteen and got married at twenty-one – far too young to know myself, let alone another person. I was very shy and tended to stay in the background, whereas he had a big personality; he was intelligent, loud and boisterous – the life and soul of the party. We had a son, and while he was young I was self-employed as an administrator. Life seemed to pass by in the usual daily round. The relationship with my husband was not a healthy one for either of us and the marriage ended after twenty-three years. It was his choice to be with someone else at that time. I'd been with him my whole adult life. I was forty-three and in deep shock – it took me years to even venture out of the house except for work. On reflection it was a positive turning point in my life, but that's only with the benefit of hindsight.

Not long **before** my marriage ended, my mother and brother died within ten days of each other. It was a terribly unhappy and traumatic time for the whole family, but we were very lucky that we could talk, cry and grieve for our losses together. We helped each other through the hurricane that their deaths visited upon us.

After these personal tragedies I was washed up for about three years. But on my forty-sixth birthday my sister and my friend said, 'Right – we are going out!' I really didn't want to go, but they made me, and we went to the nearest place, which was a Wetherspoons. But it didn't matter – it sold wine. It's perhaps not the scenario you might imagine for a transformative experience, but I met someone that night and we got on very well, although he was a lot younger than me. I didn't see him again for several months but I think a tiny spark, which had been kindling, was ignited within me.

Slowly I gained confidence. I laughed a lot and felt attractive. I started to teach myself to own my life, to take charge of my life and to see it as an opportunity and an adventure. I knew I had to make changes and so I started trying out new things. I read a huge number of self-help books. Susan Jeffers's *Feel the Fear and Do It Anyway* really resonated. I began to see everything as learning, rather than polarising things into good and bad or success and failure. I decided to do some things that would challenge me. I hadn't been on holiday without my husband since I was fifteen; I decided if I was going to do it, I'd do it big-time, and I set my sights on a touring holiday in Australia. I went with my teenage son and my sister to Australia for three weeks and it was a really big deal for me. I organised it all and was so proud that the arrangements ran smoothly. I managed to conquer my fear of being single and taking responsibility. We had a great time, climbing Sydney Harbour Bridge, snorkelling on the Great Barrier Reef and walking around Uluru, which took five hours in sweltering heat. The trip reassured me that I could cope, and it was an important thing for me to recognise in myself.

It's taken me twenty years since coming out of an unhealthy relationship to build my confidence. I married far too young and knew so little about life. I sometimes lament not having been a wild teenager who got the chance to learn by my mistakes.

I began to set myself new challenges and, more importantly, to enjoy life. I tried out many things and took a few courses; the one I enjoyed most was Practical Philosophy, run by the London School of Economics, which had satellite groups all over the country. The group in Manchester was brilliant, with a lovely set of students and a great teacher. It helped me to understand not only myself but also how to handle life. The mantra of the class was 'What would a wise person do?' and I ask this question regularly – it never fails to help me. I went on to study philosophy for several years.

Without that course I'm not sure I would have had the sureness to make the decisions I later made. I attended an arts festival at Waterperry Gardens near Oxford, where environmental activist

Satish Kumar spoke about trusting that the universe will provide. His talk helped me realise that anything is possible and that I could cope – this led me to start paring things back, trying to be simply present to internal (and external) minimalism. I began the practice of trying not to overcomplicate things in my head – not to control or worry about the future, but to accept that all would be just as it should be, however that turned out.

This led to my learning to meditate, and it was during this period of reflection that my thoughts led me to my big move. It didn't happen in a straight line. I had a couple of relationships, one with a football coach who now lives in America. I visited, with the idea of maybe moving there, but decided it wasn't for me.

I made a new group of friends who were my age and who were real party animals. There I was, almost fifty, having not been 'out there' much since I was fifteen, thinking, 'Wow, party-time!' I went to festivals, stayed out late, and 'came in with the milkman'. The morning I literally came in with the milkman I thought, 'Yes, I'm a rebel.' I did a lot of great stuff and had an absolute ball – it was an exciting time for me, for the exuberant, fun, laid-back side of me that I'd never had chance to explore. But eventually I knew that I couldn't carry on with this lifestyle. Sex, drugs and rock-'n'-roll are some of the things I should have experienced as a teenager. As an older woman, I needed a change.

Slowly I started to plan a move away from the Manchester area. It was all I'd ever known. It was my birthplace, and my whole family and good friends were there. But as with all relationships it was complicated, and I felt that I wanted a fresh start. I did it all in a measured, step-by-step way, as I wasn't sure what I was going to do. I didn't talk about it with family or friends. I changed my job, sold my house, and moved into rented property so that if I wanted to move or do something different I was well placed. I put a series of little things in motion, ready for my big leap. Selling the house was the biggest step in 'letting go'. I was no longer attached to the house, and that taught me not to attach to other things. I can't put into words how liberating that was. Some people were upset that I was making big changes. It may have been out of fear that they were losing a friend, someone to have a good time with.

Around that time, on a trip to Cornwall, I got off the plane in Newquay and went to meet my son and his wife and friends on Perranporth beach. It was a beautiful evening, there was a gorgeous sunset, and people were having barbecues on the beach. I thought, why wouldn't I want to do this every day? And I realised that I was the one who could make that choice. I was fifty-nine by then. When I returned to Manchester, I gave notice at my job at the Clinical Research Centre and on my rental property. I moved to Cornwall just one month later. I think I had put everything in place to allow myself to do this. I wanted something *to* happen and I had arranged my life so that something *could* happen. When I left for Cornwall, everyone said, 'Wow, that's a sudden, rash decision', but it wasn't really. I was steady in my approach and I'd prepared myself practically and emotionally for it.

My fears about getting work were heightened by well-meaning friends telling me that I'd never get a job in Cornwall at my age. But I did. Because of my experience, the university welcomed me to their administration team. With dwindling funds and a desire to stay in Cornwall, I bought a mobile home in need of some TLC. It was a project, but now it's a perfect 36ft by 10ft home on a residential site in a lovely valley. Now I know that I can live with less than before,

I prefer it. I eventually bought a long-searched-for VW campervan too, so I had the best of both worlds – a home base and a home-from-home to do some travelling in.

Once I'd moved to Cornwall I felt like a different person. I enjoyed being on my own; I'd always been in the background but now I was starting to feel stronger, living in the knowledge that I was going to be OK. That inner sense is so vital, so empowering. Cornwall has become an adventure playground for me. I've put myself out there. When I arrived here, I volunteered for South West Water, planting trees and clearing ponds and helping with outdoor activities at BF Adventure, a children's charity. I can't read music and I'm not a great singer, but I joined a choir and quickly got involved with Wildworks, an outdoor community theatre group. There's nothing quite like singing outdoors, especially in settings like The Lost Gardens of Heligan, Trelowarren Estate and Porthmeor Beach. It's been a wonderful experience and I've built a lovely group of friends here. The first time I was in Falmouth and someone said 'Hi', I felt like I'd started to belong.

I've trained myself to say 'yes' to everything and if I don't like it, I just don't do it again. I've started sea swimming with a group of friends and I'm now swimming in the winter (in a wetsuit). It's exhilarating! I did a Christmas Day swim in just my costume, with hundreds of other swimmers. It was freezing, but the energy of the group embraced me.

Soon after moving to Cornwall, I attended a couple of funerals which I found really upsetting because of the lack of care taken over them. One was for an eighty-six-year-old lady – she had had a long, interesting and eventful life that wasn't celebrated at all. I left the funeral feeling saddened that her life – her achievements, her sorrows, her loves – weren't recognised. She deserved more, and I was sure there was a better way of acknowledging a life.

I think that when we're receptive, serendipity can be a wonderful ally. I heard a fellow choir member mention that she was a celebrant, so I asked her a lot of questions. I was noticing, curious, seeing the world and myself with fresh eyes. I began to research what being a celebrant involved. More and more it began to feel like 'me'. Like most people, as they get older, I'd started to think about my own mortality; what would happen and what did it mean for me? The more I thought about the funerals I'd attended, the more I thought that I could do better. For someone who's shy and has never liked public speaking, this was a bold idea. I researched it well and gave myself plenty of thinking time. It felt like it was meant to be. Then came the jumping-off-the-ledge point – I could continue thinking indefinitely or I could just get on and do it.

I researched a few celebrant trainers and found Veronika Robinson's 'heart-led' training, which resonated with me. A heart-led celebrant creates, writes and officiates ceremonies with integrity, acceptance and creativity, which is exactly how I wanted my role as celebrant to be. At that time, working for the university, I had the benefit of a long summer vacation. If I didn't do it then, while I had that gift of time, I might never do it. In 2019 I set off in Bessie, my campervan, for the northwest again, this time to Carlisle, to start my training.

Celebrancy goes beyond what has traditionally been seen as the trilogy of religious ceremony: births, marriages and deaths. It includes those ceremonies, but extends to all rites of passage that are significant and meaningful to community – a naming ceremony for a child, connecting them to family, friends and forebears; a ritual at times of separation, allowing acceptance and the setting of intentions; a vow renewal to strengthen a partnership or move a relationship into a new phase of life; or a memorial ceremony which can be held many months after a death, supporting acceptance or allowing the celebration or recognition of life. As part of my training I was asked to write my own eulogy. It was challenging and a little unnerving. Sometimes we don't see our lives as significant and we focus on shortcomings, on this mistake or that limitation, or on a catalogue of difficult life events such as divorce, accidents and bereavements. With a tendency to focus on the ordinary rather than the extraordinary, we can overlook the creative ways we have overcome life's challenges, or the serendipitous, wonderful things we've done or that have happened to us.

It was a great privilege for me to be able to help a friend reframe the view she had of her life by writing her eulogy. She provided an original draft and, when I read it, I was shocked at the bleak interpretation of her story. I've always seen her as strong, resilient, generous, adaptable and determined. I reframed her life story by focusing on how she had surmounted many trials and on the great friendships she had formed because of the events she had experienced. I didn't change anything except the viewpoint. When she read it she said, 'Wow, put like that it sounds like a life worth living.' This strong-minded woman continues to show her strength in living with cancer.

Another joy has been in having three of my rituals published in *The Celebrant*, an international journal for celebrants and ceremonies. It was thrilling and encouraging to see in print something I had written. I've also started to learn British Sign Language; I'd like to be able to welcome all people and introduce myself at a ceremony.

A question arose during my training that challenged me for quite a while: 'Do you believe in marriage?' To deliver a meaningful service you must believe in the ceremony you are performing. It took me quite a while to have an honest conversation with myself and I concluded that, yes, I do believe in marriage. I believe in love. I accept that not every marriage is going to last, as in my own case and millions of others, but the starting point is love, and that is what I believe in. Of course, the real challenge is that weddings tend to be planned years in advance, and while I'm growing as a person on this voyage of discovery, I can only imagine what Juicy Crone adventures I'll be up to in two years' time. But I can be discerning about which ceremonies I would like to share in. That's one of the things about being a crone – I've learned that the word 'no' can be my friend too. So, if it's next week, next month or next Christmas, I will delight in celebrating true love.

After I completed my training, I was excited and ready to go, but I needed to keep my feet on the ground. I have modest means and I needed to make sure I could continue to look after myself financially. I took a business course to learn about self-employment, tax, record keeping, my professional responsibilities and so on. My confidence grew and I was poised to launch myself as an independent celebrant.

After lockdown restrictions eased, I was the celebrant at several funerals. It's such a privilege to be present for bereaved families and to tell the meaningful life story of the person who has died. It's affirming when a family member says, 'Mum would have loved that. I could really see her.' (And a thank-you gift of a rather good single malt whisky was unexpected but very welcome!) My dream is that one day we will all be able to talk about death if we choose to, for it not to be a taboo subject. Our culture removes us from it, yet it's the surest thing in our lives.

Someone once said to me, 'I don't know how you do it', and I don't know how I do it either. The younger me could never have imagined being confident enough to stand up and lead in this way. But in the doing, it feels absolutely like me – wanting to create a better, more meaningful experience. The listeners may all be looking at me (which I'm not comfortable with yet), but it's not me they're focusing on. If I'm doing things right, they're remembering the person they're saying goodbye to, listening intently to a couple's love story, or appreciating the significance in bestowing a name.

The celebrancy training was a rite of passage, too. Although it sounds counter-intuitive, there's an enormous richness in pondering the existential questions surrounding death, dying and love. I feel that my life has been enriched and enhanced by reflecting on these themes. It's part of my transition into the wisdom years and my transformation as a woman. I'm nervous about it; I want to be prepared for my own death, to accept it as best I can. I do everything I can to keep myself fit and well. I walk, swim, sing. But of course, none of us knows the shape of things to come. Those thoughts and feelings have collided with the huge existential questions that Covid has presented. Accepting the not-knowing is a difficult but essential part of finding happiness.

Life in Cornwall continues to throw up opportunities and challenges. A fellow gardener invited me to join other women at a Beltane celebration at the Bronze Age Boscawen-Un stone circle. The pagan festival of Beltane falls on May Day, halfway between the spring equinox and the summer solstice. I was intrigued and a little nervous – it sounded a bit 'hippy' – but it was wonderful. Rituals greeted us gathering together – we lay in a circle, focusing on the sacred space we held under a perfect evening sky. We meditated on the body chakras, in particular the sacral chakra. We created a sort of maypole using the scarves everyone had brought and then we danced. We danced, as the saying goes, 'like no-one was watching' through the ancient stones until the sun went down. I hadn't danced like that for years. I felt uninhibited. I let go of my inner censor telling me I was sixty-four and shouldn't be doing this. It was uplifting and empowering. Afterwards we came together in a circle of contemplation around the fire while we listened to a harpist playing.

We shared our thoughts about the evening and how it had made us feel as women. It was the first time I had verbalised my feeling of loss when my periods had stopped and I realised I was beyond childbearing. I was forty-six when that happened, and somehow I felt that I'd lost a huge part of my being a woman. I felt free to talk about it there. I expressed the sense of feeling less sexy with the passing of time. I couldn't have received a more positive, life-affirming reaction from this group of women, most of whom I'd never met before, supporting everything I now had to offer others, the community, and myself.

At times I've sought out things which I've then found I no longer feel comfortable with – belly dancing, for instance. It occurs to me that by stepping back into the activities of younger years, of youth and energy, I'm not being present in the absolute joy to be had in the moment. *This* is my time to be sixty-five. This might mean learning how to belly dance, but I have a sense that I'm on the cusp of something more profound, and that by trying to regain my youth I'm jeopardising the richness of what is happening in the here and now.

I do sometimes still get a sense of being edged to the periphery, but it's at those times that I'm galvanised into a determination not to disappear from my own life. I intend to live every day as my best self.

My crone years have enabled me to claim myself; it takes a lot of work and self-reflection to get to a place of self-acceptance. I don't carry my past, but I'm grateful for all it has shown me. I've learned what it means to be 'happy to sit in one's own presence'. It's a wonderful feeling to know I'm OK. I am accepting of my past and am at peace with it. I truly no longer feel that I have a hole in my heart, physical or metaphorical. I know what my heart is telling me, and I have the wisdom, the courage and the energy to follow it.

17

SUPRIYA'S STORY: BOMBAY TO BJÖRK

Singing has an immediate and unpredictable impact. As soon as sound is pouring out of your mouth, you are brought into the present moment, face to face with yourself, and there is nowhere to hide. It's like falling in love.

Chloë Goodchild, *The Naked Voice*

The work of Barbara Hepworth moves me deeply. I had been to see her work in St Ives and the Yorkshire Sculpture Park, but when I arranged to meet Supriya at the latter, as it was near her home, I did not know that Hepworth and the park were very close to her heart too. It was one of those endearing serendipitous moments of connection.

Supriya and I spent the morning together in the sculpture park café, working our way through several courses of brunch, cups of coffee and pots of tea as she told me her story. Hers was one of the last interviews I conducted for this book and her tale added to my respect and amazement at the tenacity, creativity and sheer joyfulness of crones. Having spent so many warm and candid moments with Supriya, I was sorry to have to say goodbye. As I left Yorkshire and headed south, I reflected that she has embraced every stage of her life, including this third act, with gusto. Since then I have enjoyed following her career on social media – from traditional concert venues to churches to festivals such as Womad. So Björk, if you are listening, please get in contact with Supriya. Have a Carnatic experience for yourself, and make her dream come true!

I was very fortunate to be born and brought up in Mumbai (formerly Bombay), the cultural and financial capital of India. My father was an auditor and we lived in government quarters in a high-rise apartment block of some forty households. I learned six or seven languages, and so much more, from all the families in my quarters. I had a fabulous childhood. My brother was eleven years older than me and I was a much longed-for second child.

Like most children of my generation, I lived my life outdoors, playing with friends and exploring. I didn't spend much time on schoolwork because everything else was much more interesting. For me, school was about friends. I have always loved people and socialising – the world is full of human beings and I find them fascinating. I loved all my extra-curricular activities, especially music and dance.

Left to my own devices I probably would have pursued my fascination with the human mind, perhaps studying psychiatry, but I didn't know that about myself then. It was assumed that I would follow my father and my brother, who was an accountant, into a career in finance. My parents' wishes counted for a lot and I would never have disappointed them.

I studied at Bombay University for a degree in commerce and accountancy, but again it was the extra-curricular activities that I enjoyed the most. I even played for the university's women's cricket team – this was before women's cricket was heard of.

After I graduated, a friend of the family, who had a connection at HSBC (Hongkong and Shanghai Banking Corporation), suggested that I give her my CV. I did so, and was invited to sit the entrance exam. HSBC was computerising its entire banking system at the time and needed extra staff to set up the system. Everyone was thrilled that I was offered a job – it was seen as a prestigious and exciting opportunity to work for a foreign bank – but it bored the life out of me; with the confidence of youth I thought I could get a better position. One day I went to a senior manager and told him that I was quitting, but that he should contact me if a more interesting role became available. I then went out to the movies with a friend. I still cannot believe myself! Sure enough, a few weeks later I was invited for interview for a job in Human Resources, a job that really engaged me. This taught me that if you don't ask, you don't get. I have taught my daughter the same: the worst that can happen is that they say no.

Soon afterwards, my mother raised the question of choosing a marriage partner for me. I could not have imagined selecting my own groom. I was born a Tamil Brahmin. Being born into this caste came with both privilege and responsibility. For me it meant being well versed in the Vedas (Hindu scripture), academic achievement and time spent in philosophical reflection – looking deeply at life, nature and spirituality. And of course my parents wanted me to marry someone from that community. I stipulated that I didn't want anyone who smoked or drank, and he had to be well educated. I continued working in Mumbai for two years. One day my mother told me she had been approached by a very nice family and had found Raja for me. He was a doctor (of course he was!), a nice man from a good family, and would I like to meet him? I agreed in a half-hearted way, feeling sure that I would say no. I was happy as I was, and really enjoying my job. But then, to everyone's surprise (including mine), I fell in love.

In keeping with tradition we were married three months later. We got to know each other after we married and, do you know, it works – if you have the will to make it work. He was – he *is* – a very sweet man, very straightforward. Yesterday was our thirty-third wedding anniversary. We have faced life's challenges together. I see marriage as sailing a boat together; you are in the same vessel, on the same sea, and need to navigate the weather as it happens – storms, sunshine, and being becalmed.

After we married I followed Raja to where his work and family were, in Chennai (formerly Madras) in eastern India. Fortune favoured me again and for the first time in its history the bank transferred an employee from Mumbai to Chennai. I worked during both of my pregnancies and my career continued to thrive. There followed several years of trying to establish ourselves and build a secure base for our growing family.

Some of Raja's friends had moved to the UK to work for the NHS and we decided that we should try a similar move. At first Raja travelled alone, starting a job in Worcester, and then I was offered the chance to attend the HSBC training centre in Bricket Wood, Hertfordshire. It was a beautiful place, with over a hundred acres of landscaped grounds and facilities, used for training employees from seventy-six countries. After the training I returned to Mumbai while Raja continued working in the UK. My new role was to set up the credit card system in India. It was a huge job, with a lot of travelling and responsibility. The children were very young and my parents stepped in to help with childcare. I decided that my children wouldn't go to school for that year – I wanted them to play and to learn from my parents. Education in India is very combative and pressured and I didn't want to expose them to that before it was necessary. I wanted my children to explore the things they loved and have a liberal education. Even then I was very Scandinavian at heart! (Later, with my music, I learned how much of an affinity I feel with all things Scandinavian.)

My mother then suddenly became ill, and died shortly afterwards. I was devastated. It was the turning point in my life. The human mind has a protective membrane; it is unable to accept that someone we love so much will die. It is inconceivable. We made difficult life choices and I decided to move with the children to England. We wanted the best for our children, and England was a natural choice for us. By emigrating we would be able to give them a better chance at both education and life. The competition and school reservation system in India means that as Brahmins our children would be expected to score ninety-nine percent in their exams to get anywhere. The successful medical career my daughter Divya and son Vikram have built would not have been possible as easily in India.

We landed at Heathrow in 1997, wearing flip-flops! Raja was there to meet us, and we took the train to Worcester. That evening is still clear in my mind. We arrived at nine o'clock at night and it was still sunny. I had never lived with seasonal change; the children refused to go to bed because it was still light, and they wanted to play outside. They attended local schools and we lived in NHS staff accommodation for a while.

When I was in India I spent a lot of my salary on books. I'm a very inquisitive person; I need to know everything about the world. I found that I absolutely loved English libraries – I couldn't believe that all these books were there for us to borrow, free of charge. We all read voraciously and I took the children there two or three times a week – it was a wonderland. I read anything and everything, from Shakespeare to pulp fiction.

HSBC offered me a job in Stourbridge, in the West Midlands, as a customer service manager. HSBC data centres were being formed at the time, and this gave me a glimpse into what the future of the bank might look like. When Raja become a family doctor, a general practitioner (GP), we moved to Wigan and then to Jersey, and finally Raja moved to a GP practice in Yorkshire where we settled and bought our first house in England. The children had been to six primary schools in almost as many years.

We had been striving for so long as a family that it was only in this space of calm water that I began to see the image of myself in the future as a sixty-year-old banker and to realise that this was not what I wanted to do for much longer. I hadn't hit menopause, but I was questioning my life.

Listening to and performing music, and in particular Carnatic music, was my happiest place. Carnatic music is the ancient classical music of southern India, evolved particularly from the Samaveda tradition, and is heard all over the southern states, including Karnataka, Andhra Pradesh and Kerala. Most importantly it was untouched by the Persian invasion, so it remains pure, and is often devoted to the Hindu gods Krishna and Rama. It is usually performed by a small ensemble and is mostly a vocal, lyrical tradition. Apart from its innate beauty, Carnatic music can lift the soul to the blissful state of Mukti, the state of enlightenment. My mother studied as a Carnatic singer and earned her diploma, but she never took it up as a profession – that was frowned upon in her time. She did, however, teach me a great deal while I was growing up – how to sing traditional Carnatic music and how to play the veena, an ancient Indian string instrument similar to the sitar. I also had two wonderful gurus in India who gave me all the musical knowledge I needed – firstly Shrimati Parvathy Krishnamurthy and later Shrimati T R Balamani.

Finally having our own home in England gave me the space to return to this love of Carnatic music and to the practice of playing and vocalising. It took me time to gain confidence and skills but I just knew it was what I wanted to do. Slowly, I wondered if it could be the start of a new career for me – to share and celebrate Carnatic singing through local schools and communities – though it was neither a logical nor a safe choice. I had no idea then how my passion might grow into a business.

A guru who I really respected and who knew Sanskrit suggested I call my new venture Manasamitra. 'Manasa' means mind or heart, and 'Mitra' means friend – friend of the heart and mind. I really love this concept. So Manasamitra was born. Only then did I realise that no-one in the UK knew what Carnatic music was and that I would have to spread the word. The only business model I knew was from my work in the bank, so I created two thousand leaflets and posted them to arts centres and schools, offering them Carnatic workshops. A week went by and I was excited, expecting to get replies taking up the offer. There was not one response. I sat in my rocking chair and realised I'd have to go back to basics and understand the industry differently; the bank sold products, but in the music industry you are selling an experience. I now know my first approach would never have worked.

The first five years of Manasamitra were an uphill struggle. I was unknown as a musician and Carnatic singing was unheard of. Not only that, but it seemed no-one was interested in understanding the music. I was confident in my abilities, but who would give me a chance?

As with all good stories, my luck began in the most unlikely of places: the Yorkshire Sculpture Park (YSP) near Wakefield. The park tended to be regarded as a place for white middle-class dog-walkers, surrounded by a large Asian diaspora who never visited it. I used to come and walk around this beautiful place and admire the work of Barbara Hepworth and the other sculptors and wonder why I didn't see anyone else who looked like me? So I approached Anna Bowman, curator of the National Arts Education Archive at the YSP. I proposed a series of events in the park that would appeal to Asian families, to be held every second Sunday in the month over the space of a year. I reached out into the diaspora and encouraged people to come, to know that the park was a place for them, too. This was the first time I had tested myself, talking the talk and walking the walk. Sometimes I performed and sometimes I invited other artists and curated programmes. It was very successful and began to change the narrative about who the YSP was for. From then on things started to take off. Manasamitra began to evolve and grow in ways that excited and challenged me. Unexpected opportunities came along and mostly I embraced them.

In 2009 we delivered a big event – the Festival of India – in York's National Railway Museum. Various opportunities came as a result, but I was still firmly in the 'diaspora' box. I was starting to feel restless – no-one outside the Asian community was interested. I'm an older Asian woman trying to get into a world of music dominated by white, Western men. Just because I look like this – a middle-aged, brown woman – doesn't mean I am defined by it. I felt I needed to wear a placard: 'I like Björk' (and bits of Bollywood, too). I needed to look outside the box I had been drawn into.

My friend Maggie McEwan helped me with my first application for Arts Council Funding. When the bid was successful, I asked her to come on board as my business development manager, which she did for a year and a half, to help us get started. Then came an intense period of making Manasamitra work as a company. It was Maggie who pointed out to me that I had left the bank in order to sing and write music and now I was sliding back into being a manager, delivering workshops, managing artists – but not doing the things that gave me personal satisfaction. Accepting this insight, I reconfigured Manasamitra to function more effectively as a business. Looking back I can see that I was on the cusp of change both physically and emotionally, and I think that helped me accept Maggie's advice, to make a choice that supported my needs. Everyone has strengths and weaknesses, and I chose from then on only to work with my strengths – I can always find someone who can do the things I'm not good at or don't enjoy or just don't want to do. Why would I waste time striving to do something that someone else is far more able to do than me? This released me to network and to perform my art, the two things I love and thrive on.

When I am singing, I connect to the spiritual world around me. As I am a practising Hindu the lyrics, the notes and the melodies all speak to me – to my soul or god within. I am a synaesthete, and music connects me to all my senses; everything matters and my music is a reaction to my total sensory experience – for example, smells become words and shapes. I draw down on this in my performances.

In terms of physicality the most important sound comes from the diaphragm, and that's why posture is so important. I sit cross-legged, as in a yoga pose, and the sound comes from that area just below the heart to deep in the belly. This applies to both lower and higher notes – it's not about having a neck or throat voice. My diaphragm is the core, the centre of my being, and it has to be ready to sing for three or four hours or more. Singing from this centre is like a meditation, a spell-like connection when the words and sounds occupy the space within and without. When I have finished, it's like coming out of a trance – my brain is fully rested. Every time I sing it is as if I have given my brain a spring clean. Many people have told me I have a young voice, and it is a gift that I don't take for granted – I hear it inside myself. It is very important to me that my voice presents in a certain way. Through it I seek to convey stories and emotions and it is important that I carefully modulate the voice as I sing so that the right elements are emphasised.

Somehow, I have a Scandinavian soul, born within a Tamil Brahmin woman. In 2013 I received a small grant (which I subsidised) to travel to Scandinavia in order to explore working there. Scandinavia changes my relationship with self. Being there becomes an ineffable experience – though for telling my story I realise that doesn't help the reader! I hear more music in the stillness. The vast open beauty of the landscape evokes a spiritual pathway that I'm still walking on. Having grown up in the hustle and bustle of a big metropolis like Mumbai, I think the stark, bleak silence appeals to my soul. It's a path I tread with reverence.

I fell in love with Norway immediately. After that initial trip, my first opportunity there was in 2016 with the Oslo Ultima festival; it all came about over a cup of tea, thanks to the vision of festival director Lars Petter Hagen. I was then introduced to the Iceland Symphony Orchestra by the Artistic Director of Airwaves (a festival in Iceland) to discuss a collaboration. The Director and Education Manager wanted to introduce diversity into the orchestra, wanted the community to experience this richness. I admired them tremendously as they worked with great strength and passion. I suggested working on the concept of lullabies; there's a commonality across the globe of wanting to soothe our children, to lull them to sleep. This developed into an immersive musical experience for children and parents alike. However old we are, we all need a lullaby from time to time. We performed 'Lullaby' in small communities and schools across Iceland, culminating in a concert in the magnificent Harpa hall in Reykjavik, to me the most beautiful concert hall in the world. I made nine trips to Reykjavik on this project and loved it more each time. Iceland and Icelanders will always be in my heart.

Since then 'Lullaby' has evolved creatively; sound artist Duncan Chapman has collaborated with us, enhancing the night-time sounds to include cicadas, nightjars and soft falling rain. We have performed the piece across the UK, including in an intimate setting within the Royal Albert Hall. That happened because I invited the CEO for coffee and explained what I had in mind. I thought it would be wonderful to perform there. I remembered my mother's advice: it's always worth asking – the worst they can say is no.

I have had to explore within myself the tension between being born as a woman into a privileged caste in India, and then seeing positive discrimination favouring the traditional lower castes and discrimination against the Brahmins. Hopefully we are just in a time of transition. When I came to England my family was welcomed, yet we experienced prejudice too. I realise that I need to spend time in self-reflection. Which of these prejudices around sex, gender, colour, religion and age have I internalised and used against myself? I often feel that I need to over-deliver, over-promise and overcompensate, because I pay too much heed to being an older Asian woman.

In 2018 I received a commission from an international festival to compose a twenty-minute piece. I said to my business manager, Jacqueline Greaves, 'It's lovely, as a brown older woman, to get commissioned for this.' She turned to me and responded, 'What makes you say that? They have given Supriya Nagarajan a commission, they haven't given an "older, Asian woman" a commission! Why are you saying that?' She's right. I'm doing myself a disservice; I get drawn into the narrative of self-doubt; am I here because I am a brown woman or because I am a good musician? Sometimes it's hard for me to get past that. I know I have been very fortunate to have a mother who believed in me and supported me to forge a career in the bank. My husband has been my biggest champion and supporter – at heart he is a feminist (with a few residual hints of Asian male!). My children keep me grounded and are also my biggest critics – but with a lot of love.

I now have my own radio show on Worldwide FM, and am happy to have carved a position for myself there, reaching a wide audience. This is where I have found happiness, balancing what fulfils me with the needs of my family, who are central to my life. I have also set up a mentoring programme for emerging female composers who are interested in cross-cultural and fusion music. I remember only too well what it was like when I was starting out. I hope these women will benefit from my experience of pitfalls and successes over the last fifteen years and will go on to have rewarding careers fulfilling their talents and passions.

The Covid pandemic, although frustrating at times, gave me space to reflect on who I am and what I want, as well as on the finite length of life. It taught me to say no – I now say no to work that I may want to do but which I know will overstretch me. If people genuinely want to work with me, they will come back – it has taken me several years to reach that place. And I now recognise when people are using me to tick some kind of 'colour' box, and know that I can say no to that, too. I no longer do huge amounts of work for little money – it's not about the money, it's about self-respect. I balance the reward, whether that's financial or personal experience, and I make a choice.

I am a dreamer. For me life is a series of possible future visions. Although they start as dreams, they are very real in my mind, and without them I would not have approached the Iceland Symphony Orchestra or the Royal Albert Hall. For me, the dream has to be big because the journey towards it is so exciting. You have to enjoy the travel as much as the destination, and you meet wonderful people along the way. So, I'm putting it out there that my big dream is to work with Björk!

We all enter and leave the world alone. Ultimately our most important relationship is with ourselves. Only recently have I been able to listen to myself without critiquing too harshly. I even enjoy my music sometimes! I have also realised that I can sing *myself* a lullaby – that it is important to give to myself what I can give to others. Music is healing and fills me with a sense of wholeness.

18

TAMSIN'S STORY:
BOIL. ZEBRA. FEAST.

…I suspect that the mind, like the feet, works at about three miles an hour. If this is so, then modern life is moving faster than the speed of thought, or thoughtfulness.

Rebecca Solnit, *Wanderlust: A History of Walking*

Eighteen months into the Covid pandemic, Tamsin sent me the what3words app coordinates for our meeting place on the coast near her home in Edinburgh: boil.zebra.feast. As it happens, my face mask has zebras on it, so I ruminated on the random – or serendipitous – nature of existence as I walked towards our meeting place.

The what3words concept is based on the mathematical notion that the world can be divided into 57 trillion squares, each measuring three square metres, and allocates each square three random words. It helps that the English language includes more than 171,000 words, although forty thousand words is, apparently, enough to create the unique combinations required to cover the globe.

As Tamsin and I walked, talked and enjoyed a luxuriously long alfresco brunch, it occurred to me that our stories are a bit like this. Life assigns us unique and sometimes seemingly random combinations. Understanding the connections between them and making sense of who we are is our life's work. Much of our talk was about how much value we place on making meaning out of serendipity and how much we questioned the certainty of black and white.

Often, we may start with a *boil*, but for those who put the work in, life can often end with a *feast*. The *zebra*? Well, we all have one of those lurking in a cupboard, don't we? As we talked, Tamsin remembered that she was conceived in Africa and that actually a zebra seemed apt as her motif. We said our goodbyes, musing on the Daoist philosophy that everything is connected, even if at first it might appear as just three random words: Boil. Zebra. Feast.

I was living on the periphery of my own life for the first fifty years. After the menopause I walked into myself wholeheartedly and unashamedly. I knew deep down that if I was ever to know myself with integrity and compassion, I needed to go for a walk – a very long walk.

For the last few years, I have made several secular pilgrimages, walking thousands of miles. They have all been portals into the core of my being – tramping frees my mind and stops everything being cerebral, existing only in my head. Step by step I meet acceptance: this is how things are.

In the first few minutes of my walks I need to clear my 'in-tray', thinking about texts and emails I meant to send, ticking things off the mental job list. But then, as the walk starts to lull me, a space opens and I start to reflect on the ones I love, the people I want to tell that I'm thinking of them.

As I walk, I'm aware of the transformation that takes place in my body. At the start of every walk I feel discomfort – pain, even – and need to talk myself through it: heel-ball-step, heel-ball-step. I sense every physical nuance, there's a stir in my neck, shoulders, hips, knees. It's a visceral sensation of things dropping down into my belly. It feels rather like leaves or raindrops falling. I am by nature a worrier – my mind is full of 'what if' and 'what about' and 'I should do this' and 'I ought to do that'. But all the activity in my head seems to be soothed by the rhythm of my feet – as my soles meet the earth I am literally grounding myself. Things start to shift and I feel myself rebalancing, holding everything in my abdomen. I apply mind over matter to come into my body, which might take a while if I'm upset about something. What I've been holding as worry in my head starts to feel like detritus and I often need to find a loo quite quickly!

Curiously, feeling the air on my skin heralds a process of allowing. After five minutes I enter the walk and come into myself; it sounds like a contradiction in terms, but the more I walk in an embodied way, the more I become aware of the world around me – I appreciate the beauty of the sky, the twist of a tree trunk, or the line of ants crossing the path. The beginning of the walk is usually slow, as I want to capture those moments with photographs or meditate on a view. By afternoon I walk more consistently. My comfortable daily distance is about twelve miles, depending on the terrain and weather.

It felt as if society and school – even home life – conspired to train me to be a good daughter, dutiful wife and mother, responding to everyone's call, until responding was a reflex. Religion and state, together, strongly guided the behaviour and expectations of women in those days. Our family unit was respectable – we were all pillars of the community. I went to church and Sunday School, sung in the choir, and attended the Girl Guides which gave out very powerful religious messages. The school careers adviser suggested

I get married and have children! However, as with most families, the pillars were undermined by family secrets. We were all living with my father's alcohol problem, but couldn't speak openly about it. There was a need to maintain the façade because mental health issues were not talked about. My dad and I kneeled side-by-side at the altar in church, whatever else had happened the night before.

Long-distance walking is the antidote to all that hiding and dissembling for others; I walk the path alone and, once my phone is off, I cannot respond to the world beyond that which is immediately around me. It sounds so obvious, but walking is about embodied movement. I trained as a dancer and then became a shiatsu practitioner, and for me movement is freeing – it frees my body, my thoughts and my emotions. In shiatsu theory, putting your feet on the ground rhythmically is an aspect of the earth element, which is linked to issues of self-esteem and having the wherewithal to put yourself at the centre of your life.

I am so drawn to a life of solitude that I have thought many times about joining a nunnery. I have practised Zen Buddhist meditation for many years; I am not religious, but as a spiritual practice it offers me a powerful alternative to the rigid Christianity I was brought up with. Quite apart from the insurmountable hurdle of being a non-believer, I could not leave my loved ones to enter a convent. However, knowing what my needs are, I am trying to find a balance between a solitary life and one lived with family and in society. It's not easy to maintain this in equilibrium.

After my husband left, being a single parent challenged what I thought I knew about raising children. I believed that for children to be well, they needed two parents, one of each sex. That children should be raised only in a heterosexual, nuclear family. After a while

I started to question my feelings about gender roles and my own sexuality. Walking long distances offers the opportunity to muse on the faces we present to the world. Walking for days on end I laughed at myself presenting as a boy scout in shorts, T-shirt and sun hat – yet inside I sometimes felt powerful and statuesque like the pictures of African women my parents showed me from Ghana where I was conceived.

At school, I had had feelings for another girl and we started to explore together. I remember it as a joyful experience, but for some reason I told my mother, whose response was not at all positive. She was very clear that it must never happen again, so although there were others I wanted to be with, I concealed it and felt a huge weight of shame and guilt. When, about eight years after my marriage ended, I came out as lesbian to my family and close friends, my Mum was supportive. As Gloria Steinem writes in *Revolution from Within*:

> Our sexuality is such a deep, spontaneous, and powerful part of our core identity that the conscious or unconscious need to falsify it is a little death … concealing any part of our true self is a partial death.

Since then, I've had relationships with men, and I think more about the relationship itself – is this person right for me? Regardless of their sex or gender, is there a spark? Do they have integrity? Do they make me happy? Does the relationship need a label, or can it just *be*? I am trying to understand more – I wonder if I trust myself to not be subsumed by others. Walking allows me to be solidly me, whereas in relationships I feel I can quickly get lost. It's something I'm working on – shedding the layer of conditioning that everything is dependent on what other people expect of me.

When I was in my fifties several life events collided: my children left home, I had to leave a business I had set up and put everything into, and menopause was in full swing. People talk about empty nest syndrome in such a glib way, as if giving twenty-plus years to caring for another is trivial. I sat on my soft red sofa for a year trying to make sense of my world. What was my relationship now with my grown-up children? What were my feelings about living here in the family home alone? Who was I?

The combination of these major events, followed by the death of my father, brought my thoughts back to going for a walk – a very long walk. There was a very long run-up to me going for a very long walk – fifty years, in fact. Perhaps the length of my walks has been in direct correlation with the inner world that I wanted to straighten out.

One October morning in 2016, aged fifty-three, I woke up and thought, 'I'm going to Spain to walk the Camino!' That was it. It was something I needed to do for my own survival. *Camino* means both the act of walking and path in Spanish, both of which imply a metaphysical journey; when people talk of 'the Camino', they are talking about the Camino de Santiago, a large network of pilgrim routes, totalling several thousand miles, stretching across Europe. Telling my clients and my students and my independent, grown-up children that I was leaving was a terrible wrench. Everyone seemed to feel abandoned, and they feared for my safety. It caused such a rumpus that in the end I referred to it as my 'sabbatical', which curiously was more palatable – I think it sounded masculine and academic – and people started to calm down. One elderly aunt was very supportive and slipped me fifty quid – she may never know how much strength that gave me.

I stayed on the south coast of England with my extended family, taking a few Spanish classes before I left. I took the boat from Portsmouth to Santander on my father's birthday, with all the emotional charge that entailed. The twenty-four-hour crossing gave me time to collect my thoughts. I began to sense how tired I was, and how exhausting the last few years had been, but I also felt a little bubble of excitement rising.

I knew I wanted to walk the Camino but I had planned nothing. I believe this was the most empowering thing for me after a life spent organising: list-writing, managing a family, being redoubtable at juggling and organising the household, family, work. I stopped. Had I done that for too long, perhaps? The only thing I knew was that something had to change. In complete contrast to every aspect of my life before, I followed my intuition and allowed fortune to guide me. I didn't know from one day to the next what I was going to do, only that I had promised everyone that I would be back home at the end of the year. When something presented itself, I somehow knew what to act on. I had to trust that – had to give myself over and wait. It was neither logical nor cerebral. I had to be vulnerable and step out into the unknown. By allowing that to happen I could respond in kind and accept offers of accommodation, accept helping hands and friendship when they were offered. One thing led to another and then another, it required no reaching or searching. It was the opposite of what you're expected to do when setting out on a very long trip; here I was, a post-menopausal woman, surrendering myself to a new way of being, to my intuition, to what turned out to be the practice of self-care and self-knowing.

I gave myself a month to acclimatise in Spain before I set off on the route. I built up stamina with day walks in the Pays Basque to get myself in shape and to adjust to life in a different country. Like a modern-day troubadour, I used my skills as a shiatsu practitioner in exchange for bed and board with people who I had been put in touch with by friends and colleagues. I was worried that I might not cope with the weight of the rucksack, which at nearly three stone was heavier than the recommended twenty per cent of body weight. To mitigate these concerns and my feelings of vulnerability, I decided to start the pilgrimage halfway between Pamplona and Puente la Reina, rather than from Saint-Jean-Pied-de-Port, the traditional starting point of the Camino Frances.

The Camino de Santiago is not a single long-distance footpath but a lattice of European pilgrim routes, all converging at Santiago de Compostela in northwest Spain. The paths traverse Spain, France, Portugal, Israel, England and many more territories. You will often see scallop shells – coquilles St-Jacques – dangling from the backpacks of the pilgrims, the shells' ridges symbolising the many routes which converge on Santiago.

The most common question I have been asked is about my feet! I had a week or so of blisters at the beginning, but I'd researched what to take with me before going, and had plasters, cream and a sewing kit (yes, we sew a thread through the blister and let the fluid drain out over time to stop it getting infected). The other pilgrims were helpful and showed me how to look after my feet, so I didn't have to stop. My skin hardened up soon enough.

I set off from near Pamplona feeling nervous and excited; my rucksack felt very heavy. But all that yoga before I left – my daily salutations to the sun – had helped. Dance training stood me in very good stead in tolerating the inevitable pain at the end of the first few days and the stiffness each morning. (Having said that, following this experience and before my next long walk I bought a modern, lightweight sleeping bag and towel to lighten my pack.) I used my shiatsu and other practices to identify the source of any discomfort and to relax into the areas I was holding in tension – and lo! they disappeared as quickly as they came. Gradually my muscles remembered their elasticity.

There were many other people who suffered and some who had to give up. I helped with shiatsu where I could (feet, hands, ankles, backs, etc) in the evenings at the hostels and along the path. I was pleased to meet travellers further along the way who I had given massages, particularly in Santiago on the final day, knowing they had been able to complete the hike.

The Camino route is set up for the needs of all pilgrims, whether devout or secular. *Albergues* (hostels) run by churches, local governments and non-profit organisations offer basic accommodation, usually in the form of dormitories with bunk beds, at around five euros per night (the more luxurious private accommodation is much more expensive). They are designed specifically for pilgrims and are a great place to meet new people and connect with fellow walkers.

After five weeks and 431 miles of walking I arrived in Santiago. I was elated, proud, changed. Yet almost immediately I turned around and started walking south into the mountains. I was not ready for my pilgrimage to end. I then spent another month in reflective walking in a less structured way around Madrid, Valencia and the Sierra Calderona. I felt as if there was still more, that I had more to learn from the confluence of the many paths I had trodden in my life.

I returned home in time for Christmas, as I promised I would. After three months of walking it was such a shock; I missed the life of the long-distance walker so much that I needed to return. Following three months in the UK, in March I did. I headed out to walk the Via de la Plata, or Silver Way – an ancient trade route that is also a spiritual pilgrimage, like the Camino – 620 miles from Seville to Santiago. As I walked I planned my first book: *Working with Death and Loss in Shiatsu Practice, a Guide to Bodywork in Palliative Care.* Complementary medicine is playing an increasingly important role in dying well, and I was honoured to be asked to write it. After another season at home I went to Estonia on retreat to finish the manuscript.

Over time I've found a rhythm to life that suits me. I walk for three months, come home for three months, rinse and repeat. My pilgrimages since then have found me on the Via Sacra in Austria, the Camino in Portugal, up the Alps and around the lakes of Switzerland, and, when I'm home based, the St Magnus Way on Orkney and the Fife and Berwickshire coastal paths.

In a sense we are all pilgrims; we are all travelling towards a place in the distance. We live our lives in tension between prescription and choice, and providence plays a large part in the balance of these two sometimes uneasy bedfellows. I am aware of how incredibly lucky I am as a Western woman to be able to make the choices I have made. We are all in eternal movement and I have chosen to make some of that movement through thousands of pilgrim miles. I have walked into the exploration of self – while walking I have had a passionate affair with a French man and then one with an English woman. I have made peace with the accident of my birth, my 'boil', including the trans-generational trauma which is present to a greater or lesser extent in all of us.

After my children left home, at first my moral compass wouldn't allow me to enjoy having the house to myself, so I filled it with homeless people, lodgers, couch-surfers, Airbnb guests. During the Covid lockdown, however, for the first time in my life I found myself living alone. This offered another way for me to discover who I was, and to find out more about my relationship with my home. Living alone now feels like the greatest indulgence of my life. I've slowly spread out and inhabited every room – I have shiatsu in one room, art and sewing in another. It feels naughty, self-indulgent, unkind, ungenerous, but it also feels amazing and luxurious. The reality is, however, that I will have to get a lodger to help cover my bills.

My walks in Europe were transformative; after childbirth they were probably the most powerful experiences of my life, and there are still many long-distance paths I would like to tread. I don't feel as comfortable travelling today, partly because of Covid-19 but mostly as a personal response to climate change. Lockdown gave me the space to contemplate what need is met in me by long walks and why they fill me – how can I replicate that while monitoring my carbon footprint and being mindful of this inner need as I get older? With this in mind, I've turned my attention to walking in the UK. I've started the Pilgrims Way, and in October 2021 I walked a coast-to-coast route from Dunbar to Glasgow with other pilgrims for COP26, to raise awareness of the climate and ecological crisis.

When I was walking the Camino de Santiago, I learned that it is the simplicity of the everyday that becomes the spiritual practice, an autonomic governance. Apart from food intake, rucksack contents and following the map, there is nothing else. It is immensely freeing. And yet I question myself: if this is true, then why do I feel the need to blog about it, make artwork, be visible, be heard? Perhaps that is what makes us human. People say to me, 'Oh I wish I could do that – you're so lucky (or brave, or special).' That's not true. I just couldn't *not* do it, and the more I walked the easier it was to give myself permission to do so.

I have an internal battle going on. I criticise myself for being a butterfly, for flitting from one thing to another: shiatsu, writing, art projects, sound projects, long-distance walking, my work around death. But then I think of the nature of a butterfly – it flits to feed on nectar, that's what sustains it. This is me. This is who I am. That stops the voice of the inner critic: *you're all over the place*. My flittings are my adventure, and sometimes they take the form of very long walks and sometimes a dalliance with a new experience that may last only a few seconds.

19

PEACHES AND FIGS

I'm beginning to realize the pleasure of being a nothing-to-lose, take-no-shit older woman…

Gloria Steinem, *The Truth Will Set You Free, but First It Will Piss You Off!*

I'm driving into my local market town with my van window down, glad of some fresh air after a day at my desk. I have an appointment with 'The Great Reformer' in the Pilates studio. Nestled on the Gloucestershire/Herefordshire border, the town, known for its gentle good manners and slow ways, is busy with farmers and children coming out of school. We drivers queue, wing mirror to wing mirror, nudging past each other as we progress. A couple of lads in a souped-up Audi, heading in the opposite direction, draw alongside me, music blaring. One looks at me and shouts, 'Old cunt.' I am stunned, shocked. Silent.

We used to teach primary school children impulse control with the 'Think-Act' rule. 'Stop-Breathe-Think'. Think of three responses. These are mine:

1. A hand gesture.
2. Be afraid, be very afraid – an army of white-haired witches is coming to get you!
3. Wow! You're clever, that's almost exactly what my doctor diagnosed ten years ago. I was wondering if I needed a second opinion.

Of course, he was long gone before any of this could be said or done. On the bright side, at least I no longer felt invisible. He had seen me, and I had made him angry – I've no idea why. Obviously, if misogyny were a hate crime, I would have reported the incident to the police. But this hate speech was directed at me because I am a woman, not because of the characteristics currently protected by hate crime legislation: disability, ethnicity, sexual orientation or transgender identity. I therefore don't have a legal leg to stand on.

There are more than one billion women aged over fifty on the planet, twelve million of them in the UK, and yet for some strange reason we do not own that power. We have ingested the belief that we do not hold authority, we are not influential and cannot effect change. We can, and we should. Reclaiming our wisdom years is a gift for everyone. If only there were more wisdom and less power play in the world.

My thinking has been profoundly affected by the wisdom of the many women who have contacted me and shared their stories. I have been challenged and criticised, cheered on and supported. I have mourned with them and shared their outrage at life events. I have been cared for by women I have never met in person. We have all been changed in the writing of this book. Many of the women have been encouraged and validated by taking part in this project, and for that I couldn't be happier. Together we hold out a hand and help each other along our chosen paths, we lift each other up when we stumble, and support each other when we move to a different path. And when things get tough, there's always cake. It has been the greatest honour to get to know these Juicy Crones, I am excited for them, they are doing *their thing* and that's wonderful to behold. Just as in the rest of our lives, cronehood is not a steady state. It is a place of discovery and exploration of what it means to be us.

Our third act offers us the chance of an extraordinary new way of being. It's a time of quite literally coming to our senses, of listening to our own truth for possibly the first time in our lives. Many women have told me that they feel as if they have pressed the 'reset' or 'factory setting' button and have returned to their true selves. We reassess what is important to us, we choose for ourselves which layers of our being we want to laminate, what we want to strengthen and what means of support we want in this big adventure – accepting and honouring our feelings and welcoming ourselves home to our truest self. Whether that means retreating to a reading corner for a year, paddling down the Euphrates River or playing Bingley Hall, it turns out that the strangest adventure any of us can have is an internal one, coming to an understanding of self.

One thing I welcomed as I reached my third act was also gaining a different understanding of time. In my early days of 'atrophy', I felt quite panicky, as though time were running out, and of course every day it is. None of us knows what the future holds, but statistically I had plenty of time available. The more I wholeheartedly embraced this time with new challenges and raw honesty, the more everyday experiences held huge significance for me. The division of the years into months, the days into hours, no longer has meaning. As time becomes more experiential, we are able to shift our thoughts to lived moments: those held close, treasured and wondered at. We give a place to past trauma but determine that it should not consume time or space within us – a letting go which lightens and leads. We spend time with our own fragilities and imperfections and celebrate that we can. Many of the women I talked to have enjoyed this new experience, when clock time becomes an artificial construct, and 'real' time is recorded in experiences and feelings. A lot of them told me that they had reconnected with the 'me' they were born with – the one who had somehow got lost along the way, with the passing of ordinary time. Their profound journey into cronehood was recorded in their memory as timeless because it stretched back through their whole lifetime, and that of their ancestors. They were standing in this place with the wisdom gathered throughout those years. This coming to cronehood was their whole life journey.

I am not sure if it was a moment of madness that caused me to change my name. Whatever it was, I'm blaming it on Jane Garvey, who hosted a radio discussion about the name Jane. My given name, Janice, is from the same stable and, according to family lore, if I hadn't been named Janice, I would have been a Jane or a Janet. I would have preferred Jane. I have always hated my name, and one morning before my sixty-fourth birthday I woke up and thought: why not choose a name I *do* like. So why Jay? I am not sure it's a rational choice. It just feels right. It's a coming-of-age thing. This time of my life is my time. I wanted to mark this profound stage in my life – to embrace this time as something remarkable – a rebirthing of me. Something I can hold close and celebrate, sitting on the forest floor gazing up into the canopy of ancient oaks that I often choose for company. I do feel like a whole new bird, one that has wings and can fly wherever she chooses. And I love jays, which come from the clever, cheeky corvid (crow) family. Their scientific name, *Garrulus glandarius*, meaning 'babbler of the acorns', feels apt, too. I am making my voice heard through my writing, all the while watching jays in the oak woods stash acorns away, seeding a thousand trees. With my pure white hair I smile at the thought of their distinctive, colourful attire: pinkish body, black and white markings and striking electric blue-and-black barred wings. Maybe I'll have a blue wing put in my mop to go with my new Juicy Crone name.

Changing my name was met with a mixed response. Most people accepted it immediately – 'Jay it is, then' – thank you, all. Some saw it as a sign of mental ill health, others – well, I don't really know what they thought, but it certainly made them uncomfortable. The strange thing is that when I married, aged twenty-three, and received letters addressed to 'Mrs John Smith', no-one, but no-one – except me – batted an eyelid. I had been denuded of both my names overnight and it didn't warrant a mention.

When I first conceived of writing about myself and other women who were 'free for the strangest adventures', I had a bucket list. As well as writing my first book, I wanted to travel to far-flung places, spend more time with family and friends, take long solo hikes, learn new activities, study new subjects, and so on. However long the list of things I wanted to do with this time became, I never once hovered with a pencil to add the words 'global pandemic' or indeed the crippling word 'divorce'. Yet here I am ending the writing of a book about adventure at a point when we are emerging from the Covid pandemic and I am facing life as a single woman.

I'm staying with my sister and her partner, whose house overlooks a stunning loch on the edge of the Ardnamurchan Peninsula, in northwest Scotland. They are taking wonderful care of me during this enormous time of transition. I have slept here in their guest bedroom with the incredible view better than I have slept for weeks, months possibly. What could be lovelier than being fed, held and heard by siblings when life seems to be falling apart.

I set off early one day for a short walk from their house to a favourite bay of mine. I paddle and take in as much of this wondrous place as I can, knowing that I must return home to the most painful and impossible of situations. I come here often in my dreams. It's a late August day, unusually warm for this place, but there are elements of November already practising their bass notes – there's a slight tinge to the leaves and the wind has changed its attitude slightly. This is the bay where several years before we scattered my parents' ashes. Strictly speaking, as my father and my beloved black Briard, Harry, died in the same week, there's a little of Harry in there too. Mum, Dad and huge lolloping dog, all drifting about the gulf stream. I wonder where they've been and if there is even an atom of them left in this bay. Of course, there's more than an atom of them left there for me: their presence extends to the Small Isles of Eigg, Rhum and Muck and way beyond, out to St Kilda. It is the paradise ending that they both deserved. My dad would have loved that as an adventure! I think all of us, living and dead, would be quite happy to be remembered here. The sea is crystal clear, the sand white as bones, with almost too much emotion for even this wide bay to hold. Two days previously I had swum in the bay and almost over to a small island, but I chickened out. But I'm getting braver. I might do it soon. Next year I will. There is time to emerge, to swim where the dolphins and whales are, to be out of my depth.

The granite slabs sit in purple and pink splendour, terraced conveniently so I can perch on the top, rucksack in the middle, feet on the bottom slab. My binoculars rest conveniently on a 'shelf', although I don't need to look to know that I have oystercatchers for companions. I reach for my notebook and water bottle. I've left the bottle back at the house and I do some mental gymnastics to stop me fixating on my thirst. What is it I want to say? How do I unjumble the avalanche of thoughts in my head?

A bizarre memory falls into my mind of a coach trip from junior school. With it comes a strong smell of vomit and Dettol and the sound of uncouth voices singing 'Will you still need me, will you still feed me, WHEN I'M SIXTY-FOUR?' The answer for me is apparently 'no'. This relationship that I have treasured and deferred to for twenty-five years is ending. Over the last years, while the inertia of lockdown has disabled us all, rather than find solace in each other, the gulf between us has widened. I am broken and undone. It is not what I want, but it is what I must accept. As a ten-year-old I had no notion that I would even live to be sixty-four: it was as unlikely and outlandish an idea as Sgt Pepper's Lonely Hearts Club Band.

The sea loch and bay in front of me, the backdrop of mountains, offers a glimpse of new beginnings. I feel an idea starting to form, but I have no idea what shape it might take. I have a sense of as-yet-undiscovered mysteries. My view of the small isles is giving me perspective both on my smallness and on a broader horizon. The tide opens up sandy paths to hidden islands, the ocean slides back over them, the glimpse of other worlds is lost again. A timeless sense of granite solidity, of the grain of sand of our existence and the eternity of who we are. I feel myself entering another state of being.

A grey wagtail flirts around, here, there, everywhere, nothing orderly about him. I try, like him, not to create an edifice of what my new world should, or could be like. When I finally feel ready, or have the need, to swim over to the island, I trust I will know what comes next for me, as I step into my life of solo flight.

I know that I need to find other ways of seeing and to look, to seek out the missing parts of myself. This is not a time that I was seeking, but there is luxury, a richness, to be had in retreating, pausing and reflecting. Katherine May in *Wintering* describes the process so well:

> Winter is a time of withdrawing from the world, maximising scant resources, carrying out acts of brutal efficiency and vanishing from sight; but that's where the transformation occurs. Winter is not the death of the life cycle, but its crucible.

Back at home I decide to withdraw and become an over-wintering woman. I am creating in my head a new relationship with my sense of home as a base for my solo adventure. A place for me to feel safe, to grow more hideaways in the garden, intriguing places for the grandchildren, and relaxing arbours to greet friends, old and new. I will clip the boundary hedges here and there, to allow just a glimpse of other worlds beckoning – ones yet unknown that will surprise and delight and challenge me to learn more of what it means to be a Juicy Crone. I look forward to twinkly moments of shared meaning, of surprise and of full-bellied laughter with my friends by the hearth.

I have developed a new relationship with brain fog, too. When our thinking is challenged moment by moment as we move from who we were to who we are now, it helps to think of this as making new neural pathways, which is, after all, important for learning and emotional intelligence. Putting ourselves outside our comfort zone, doing new things, helps us develop an agile brain. Not only can we be the owner-operators of our lives, but often for the first time we can control the narrative. All these women by sharing their extraordinary stories have given us hope and a little reassurance that we are, perhaps, not as mad as we may some days feel.

No amount of running or walking or singing will enlighten us if we don't observe what is going on inside of us, in the centre of our being. Sometimes confusing, often painful, usually challenging, we can, in our second spring, begin to understand our new role in the world.

For many centuries the role of the crone was integral to society, but particularly to her younger sisters. Most women relied on the wisdom of crones to heal them with herbs and plants from the hedgerow and physic garden, and to support them through the dangerous hours of labour and childbirth. During the witch trials, 'wise women' suffered and died hideously, simply because they possessed knowledge.

And yet down the years, almost as an underground movement, a crone's wisdom has endured, mother to daughter, woman to woman. We turn to our female friends for wise counsel. Never in history have there been so many post-menopausal women. We now have the weight of numbers, knowledge and power. And as older women we now have a unique opportunity to share this on a wider stage. We can reclaim the ancient status of the crone and become a force to be reckoned with. Now, more than ever we need strong, wise voices, arguing forcefully for a kind, generous and ethical approach to people and planet. By making these voices heard, we can usher in a new age of the crone.

We have all lived rich, complicated, painful and yet immensely hopeful lives. That's what makes these our wisdom years. That's what has given us permission to thumb our nose at the world and say, 'Yes, I may have wrinkles, yes, I have white hair – so what – get over yourself!' As Jamie Lee Curtis said at a 2022 conference on ageing, there has been a 'genocide of natural beauty'. We Juicy

Crones know, however, that we are wise and beautiful by any meaningful measure.

We are full of life, have a wicked sense of humour, we have honed our BS-detectors to a point of real usefulness. We can admit our mistakes and be kind to ourselves about them. I can watch my children and grandchildren grow and be that once-removed voice that can say, 'All will be well – just give it time.'

The remarkable women in this book have illustrated that this is a time that calls for courage, strength and, strangely, a trust in the power of serendipity. There have been moments while talking when each of us missed a beat and knew that something profound had happened. We may not have the cronyism of elite males on our side, but we have something so much richer – the warmth, wisdom and inspiration of our fellow crones – or cronees, as I like to think of them. A circle of cronees around us to cheer, inform and have fun with.

Perimenopause and menopause are sometimes referred to as the 'climacteric'. According to older dictionaries the 'grand climacteric' happens in the sixty-third year. I hadn't looked this word up before, but I assumed that it was related to climax – we had reached our peak and now we were on the downward slope. And indeed, the New Oxford Dictionary defines climacteric as the period of life when fertility and sexual activity are in decline. However – and this is important – some fruit, such as peaches and figs, are known as climacteric because they *improve* after they are plucked – they continue to gain in flavour and richness. Juicy Crones are definitely, I declare, a climacteric fruit. So, when you are having a bad day, just reach for a bowl of peaches and figs. Embrace the juiciness, and marinade in the goodness, depth of flavour and texture to be found there.

EPILOGUE:
HOW WAS YOUR CROSSING?

Sometimes we have to hush the frantic inner voice that says 'Don't be stupid' and learn again to look, to listen.

Kathleen Jamie, *Findings*

It's the summer of 2022 and I am on a solo trip to the Orkney islands, but my head is telling me it's 2020. That's the year I was supposed to be here – I had planned several weeks of travel around Orkney, Shetland, Iceland and the Faroes for the start of my *Juicy Crones* quest.

I have long wanted to visit Skara Brae in the West Mainland of Orkney and I am not disappointed. A Neolithic site, around 5,000 years old, it comprises a cluster of houses, complete with stone furniture which make it easy to imagine living here. At the entrance, a note informs visitors that evidence and conclusions are presented on two levels:

Printed in normal type are THINGS WE KNOW, things for which we have actual evidence based on physical remains.
Printed in italic type are THINGS WE CAN ONLY GUESS, *things that are likely* (based on what we know from elsewhere), *but for which there can be no absolute certainty.'*

This strikes me as a parallel to the wisdom we reach in our third age. That the lives we have led and the challenges we have overcome point us to understand the world more often *in italics*. All the

Juicy Crones celebrated in this book have faced life-changing events that have challenged everything they thought they knew. Their lives could no longer be written in normal type; they became uncertain of so much, of what they thought they knew, that they became italicised. Initially, living our life *in italics* can feel disorientating, sometimes frightening. However, a gradual acceptance of living with uncertainty can lead to finding unexpected pleasure, contentment even. There is a profound wisdom in those italics. They enable us to take the long view, to be less certain of what we once thought of as fact.

At Skara Brae I was made poignantly aware of other lives, lived in strong communities through countless generations and, of course, of the tiny grain of sand of my own life, and of the connections between us all. So overwhelmed was I by this sense of deep history that I needed to step away from the site for a while. There is a gate from the settlement that leads on to the Bay of Skaill. I sat there reflecting and scribbling to untangle my thoughts.

A young woman came by, and we chatted. It turned out that we were both staying on the same campsite and we met later that week for a drink. Alona is a PhD student studying island tourism on Orkney. She told me that very often when she arrives to do her research on a new island, she is asked, 'How was your crossing?' It's a question unique to those whose lives are lived via sea-roads, with all the jeopardy that entails.

It occurs to me that this is the question that needs to be asked of post-menopausal women. How was your crossing? How did you fare on the sea between your perimenopausal years and landing in this new terrain, this new post-menopausal island? It may have been calm for you – tranquil even, relatively quick; you may be one of the lucky ones who has made it across with little to remark upon. Or it may have been a stormy crossing, one on which you felt perilously close to capsizing and shipwreck or anywhere in between. However the voyage was, it will have taken years – somewhere between seven and fifteen. (Some women I spoke to reported that it took them more than twenty.) That's quite a journey – we owe it to ourselves to honour it, to ask ourselves and our fellow crones, 'How was your crossing?' To accept and celebrate that we have crossed over – that we have reached a different land, and a new life awaits us there. This recognition allows us to live life in our own unique way, unapologetically embracing our new-found island and at liberty, at last, to be 'Free for the strangest adventures'.

LISTEN

by Melanie Ward

Listen! She is calling you!
In the leap of your heart
at the sight of a star-filled sky,
in your thirst for darkness and silence.
In the deep longing that causes you
to reach out your arms and try and touch
the full moon with your heart.
She speaks to you
through whispering trees
and half-remembered dreams,
through bird-song and wolf-howl.
She wants you to know that you are
as wild, as alive and as beautiful
as the whole of Her creation.
She wants you to know that you are loved,
that you *are love*.
She longs for the truth of all that you are
just as you long for Her…
Listen! She is calling you home
to yourself.

Reproduced here by kind permission of Melanie Ward
(w wildwiseandbeautyfull.co.uk)

CRONEOGRAPHY

The following were my go-to books while I was working out what it might mean for me to live as a Juicy Crone. Some relate specifically to menopause or women's health, while others are more philosophical in nature. It's certainly not an exhaustive list – even during the short time I have been writing this book many, new books about older woman have been published. I hope it is helpful as a starting point and that you will be able to add new favourites to your own croneography.

Adichie, Chimamanda Ngozi *Notes on Grief* HarperCollins, 2021

Adichie, Chimamanda Ngozi *We Should All Be Feminists* Anchor, 2015

Albom, Mitch *Tuesdays with Morrie* Little, Brown, 2017

Atwood, Margaret *The Edible Woman* Virago, 2009

Atwood, Margaret *The Handmaid's Tale* Vintage, 1996

Baker, Sam *The Shift* Coronet, 2020

Band, Bex *Three Stripes South* Bradt, 2021

Bates, Laura *Fix the System Not the Women* Simon & Schuster, 2022

Beard, Mary *Women & Power* Profile, 2017

Beckett, Sister Wendy *Meditations on Love* Dorling Kindersley, 1996

Blackie, Sharon *If Women Rose Rooted* September, 2016

Bolen MD, Jean Shinoda *Crones Don't Whine* Conari, 2003

Bolen MD, Jean Shinoda *Goddesses in Older Women* HarperCollins 2001

Bolen MD, Jean Shinoda *The Millionth Circle* Conari, 1999

Bolen MD, Jean Shinoda *The Tao of Psychology* HarperOne, 2004

Bristol Women's Studies Group, The *Half the Sky* Virago, 1979

Brown, Brené *Daring Greatly* Penguin, 2015

Brown, Brené *Rising Strong* Penguin Random House, 2015

Bullmore, Edward *The Inflamed Mind* Short, 2019

Cameron, Deborah *Feminism* Profile, 2018

Chia, Mantak *Healing Love through the Tao* Destiny, 2005

Cleghorn, Elinor *Unwell Women* Weidenfeld & Nicolson, 2021

Codrington, Kate *Second Spring* HarperCollins, 2021

Coelho, Paulo *The Alchemist* HarperCollins, 2015

Cooke, Lucy *Bitch* Penguin Random House, 2022

Copson, Andrew & Roberts, Alice *The Little Book of Humanism* Little, Brown, 2020

Criado Perez, Caroline *Invisible Women* Penguin Random House, 2019

Csaky, Mick *How Does It Feel* Thames & Hudson, 1979

Dickinson, Emily 'My Life Had Stood a Loaded Gun' *Complete Poems* Penguin, 1933)

Dickson, Anne *The Mirror Within* Quartet, 1985

Dickson, Anne *A Woman in Your Own Right* Quartet, 1982

Dillard, Annie *The Abundance* Canongate, 2017

Dillard, Annie *The Writing Life* Harper Perennial 1990

Dinsmore-Tuli, Uma *Yoni Shakti: A Woman's Guide to Power and Freedom through Yoga and Tantra* YogaWords, 2014

Enright, Dominique *She Said* Michael O'Mara, 2018

Enright, Lynn *Vagina: a Re-Education* Allen & Unwin, 2019

Ensler, Eve *The Vagina Monologues* Virago, 2001

Estés, Clarissa Pinkola *Women Who Run with the Wolves* Ebury, 2008

Evaristo, Bernardine *Girl, Woman, Other* Penguin, 2020

Ferguson, Kirstin & Fox, Catherine *Women Kind* Murdoch, 2018

Frances-White, Deborah *The Guilty Feminist* Virago, 2019

Gates, Melinda *The Moment of Lift* Bluebird, 2019

Gladwell, Malcolm *Outliers* Penguin, 2009

Goldacre, Ben *Bad Pharma* HarperCollins, 2012

Goleman, Daniel *Destructive Emotions* Bloomsbury, 2004

Goleman, Daniel *Emotional Intelligence* Bloomsbury, 2004

Goodchild, Chloë *The Naked Voice* North Atlantic, 2015

Greer, Germaine *The Change* Penguin, 1992

Greer, Germaine *The Female Eunuch* Paladin, 1976

Greer, Germaine *The Whole Woman* Transworld, 1999

Grosz, Stephen *The Examined Life* Vintage, 2014

Heilbrun, Carolyn G *The Last Gift of Time* Ballantine, 1997

Heilbrun, Carolyn G *Writing a Woman's Life* Penguin, 1988

Hill, Maisie *Perimenopause Power* Bloomsbury, 2021

Holloway, Richard *Stories We Tell Ourselves* Canongate, 2020

Horgan, Emily & Dickson, Zachary (eds) *So Hormonal* Monstrous Regiment, 2020

Howe, E Graham *She and Me* Triton, 1974

Jacobs, Denise *Banish Your Inner Critic* Mango, 2017

Jamie, Kathleen *Findings* Sort of Books, 2005

Jeffers, Susan *Feel the Fear and Do It Anyway* Arrow, 1987

Jung, Carl *Four Archetypes* Routledge, 2003

Kennedy, Sister Stanislaus *Gardening the Soul* Simon & Schuster/TownHouse, 2001

Kenton, Leslie *Passage to Power* Vermilion, 1998

Levy, Deborah *Things I Don't Want to Know* Penguin Random House, 2014

Lewis, Helen *Difficult Women* Penguin Random House, 2020

Lewis MD, Thomas, Amini MD, Fari & Lannon MD, Richard *A General Theory of Love* Vintage, 2001

Liptrot, Amy *The Outrun* Canongate, 2016

Lister, Lisa *Love Your Lady Landscape* Hay House, 2016

Mac Cumhaill, Clare & Wiseman, Rachael *Metaphysical Animals* Penguin Random House, 2022

McGregor MD, Alyson J *Sex Matters* Quercus, 2020

May, Katherine *Wintering* Penguin, 2020

Miller, Isabel *Patience & Sarah* The Women's Press, 1979

Moran, Caitlin *More Than a Woman* Ebury, 2020

Mosconi, Dr Lisa *The XX Brain* Allen & Unwin, 2020

Nestor, James *Breath* Penguin, 2020

Nimmo, Dorothy *Kill the Black Parrot* Littlewood Arc, 1993

Oliver, Mary *Felicity* Penguin, 2015

Parks, Tim *Teach Us to Sit Still* Vintage, 2011

Pascoe, Sara *Animal* Faber & Faber, 2016

Perel, Esther *Mating in Captivity* Hodder & Stoughton, 2007

Perry, Grayson *Portrait of the Artist as a Young Girl* Vintage, 2007

Plomin, Robert *Blueprint* Penguin, 2019

Potter, Nick *The Meaning of Pain* Short, 2019

Reekie, Sandra *From YOLO to Solo* Journey Books, 2021

Reynolds Thompson, Mary *Reclaiming the Wild Soul* White Cloud, 2014

Rippon, Gina *The Gendered Brain* Vintage, 2020

Rivkin, Annabel & McMeekan, Emilie *I'm Absolutely Fine!* Octopus, 2018

Roberts, Alice *The Incredible Unlikeliness of Being* Heron, 2014

Rogers, Carl R *On Becoming a Person* Constable & Company, 1967

Ruddock, Jill Shaw *The Second Half of Your Life* Penguin Random House, 2015

Samuel, Julia *Grief Works* Penguin Random House, 2017

Samuel, Julia *This Too Shall Pass* Penguin Random House, 2020

Shepherd, Nan *The Living Mountain* Canongate, 2011

Sieghart, Mary Ann *The Authority Gap* Penguin Random House, 2021

Solnit, Rebecca *A Field Guide to Getting Lost* Canongate, 2017

Solnit, Rebecca *Men Explain Things to Me* Granta, 2014

Solnit, Rebecca *Wanderlust: A History of Walking* Verso, 2002

Sprackland, Jean *Strands* Vintage, 2013

Steinem, Gloria *Doing Sixty & Seventy* Elders Academy, 2006

Steinem, Gloria *Outrageous Acts and Everyday Rebellions* Picador, 2019

Steinem, Gloria *Revolution from Within: A Book of Self-Esteem* Bloomsbury, 1992

Steinem, Gloria *The Truth Will Set You Free, but First It Will Piss You Off!* Murdoch, 2019

Stock, Kathleen *Material Girls* Fleet, 2021

Toksvig, Sandi *Toksvig's Almanac* Trapeze 2020

Van der Kolk, Bessel *The Body Keeps the Score* Penguin Random House, 2014

Walker, Barbara G *The Crone* HarperCollins, 2015

Wallace, Christine *Germaine Greer: Untamed Shrew* Richard Cohen Books, 2000

Walters, Margaret *Feminism* Oxford University Press, 2005

Whyte, David *Consolations* Canongate, 2019

Winterson, Jeanette *Love* Penguin Random House, 2017

Wolf, Naomi *Vagina* Virago, 2013

Woolf, Virginia *A Room of One's Own and Three Guineas* Penguin Random House, 1993

Woolf, Virginia *To the Lighthouse* Penguin Random House, 2019

Yalom, Irvin D *Becoming Myself* Basic, 2017

Yalom, Irvin D *The Gift of Therapy* HarperCollins, 2010

ACKNOWLEDGEMENTS

Without all the wonderful Juicy Crones who have offered to share their stories with us, this book would not exist. More than fifty women contacted me – which was a brave and generous thing to do. Every single one of you helped me on my journey and in one way or another you have informed this book. Hearing from and meeting so many Juicy Crones has been one of the most enriching and inspiring experiences of my life. Thank you.

It was extremely difficult to choose whose story to print because they all deserved a chapter. In the end it came down to variety, offering as many versions as possible of what being a Juicy Crone might look like. To the twelve women whose stories do appear: goodness, what a journey it has been! I admire you so much for your tenacity, vulnerability, honesty and drive. I feel deeply honoured that you have trusted me with your stories – the highs, lows and deepest fears – and allowed me to retell them here. It was such a privilege to be witness to your telling, and Alex, Andie, Caroline, Deborah, Debs, Ginny, Jane, Janette, Jorj, Lesley, Supriya and Tamsin, I salute you for making your voice heard. 'Thank you' is not enough, but I do, I thank you.

All these women have worked hard to feel comfortable being a crone; all of them have given themselves permission to give birth to self, to change, grow and celebrate. If only it were as quick and painless as it sounds! We have offered each other support and wisdom and the profound reassurance that we are not alone. I now count them among my dearest friends, and I truly hope that we can continue this friendship during our journey into the unknown as 'Juicy Crones'.

One of *my* strange adventures has been writing this book. I never thought that I would be writing my first book in my mid-sixties. My heartfelt thanks go to Jean Shinoda Bolen, whose phrase 'juicy crones' made me laugh and set me on a trail to discover what it might mean. Thank you so much, Jean, for generously allowing me to use your phrase and for cheering me on to run with it. Your enthusiasm spurred me on in the bleak days when words would not flow.

Thank you to Hawkwood College in Stroud for offering a haven to rewild my soul; especially to Kevan Manwaring and Mary Reynolds Thompson who encouraged my infant steps into writing. I am deeply indebted to Stephen Moss and Gail Simmons, who not only believed in me but also encouraged me to experiment with my writing and allow my creative, somewhat subversive, nature to flourish. To my 'gang' of fellow student writers at Bath Spa University – Susie Curtin, Eleanor Halton, Richard Hibbard, Jacqui Hitt, Kelly Keegan, Hilary MacMillan, Rob Pickford and Andie Van Poeteren – thank you for your wisdom, support and fine good humour.

During the frozen months of lockdown the wonderful team at Bradt supported and encouraged my novice steps into the world of getting published. Special thanks to Adrian Phillips, who was enthusiastic about the project from our very first conversation, and to Anna Moores, whose encouragement and good humour through the bleak Covid winter even extended to sending me a mock-up of my book jacket on my lonesome lockdown birthday. Thanks also to Hilary Bradt for spurring me on and taking time to advise me: 'You will never enjoy writing any book as much as your first one, so savour it.' I have, thank you. Susannah Lord, thank you for walking me through every step of the editing process and responding to my early-morning cries for help when track changes got the better of me! My deepest thanks go to my editor, Samantha Cook. I am in awe of her skills and grateful to her many and various ways of gently nudging, suggesting and encouraging me to rewrite a passage! She has saved me from myself in more than one place with observations that made me laugh out loud – 'The jeans and the legs don't *quite* add up to an image of Moses,' she said of my description of the Queen's Guide to the Sands! Thanks Sam!

Thank you to pop artist Laura Greenan, who somehow managed to translate the ideas floating in my head into the splendid cover design. I love it, thank you. And to Melanie Ward, thank you for allowing me to include your moving poem 'Listen' – it captures so well this time in a woman's life.

To all my friends for their love, support and gentle challenges. I will not list you for fear of leaving someone out. You know who you are and I hope you know how much I value our friendship. There are some friends who have been my rock over recent months. Always there when I needed a shoulder, a laugh, or a rant: Di and Janette, thank you for your wise counsel – I don't know what I would have done without you. Ginny and Rob, thank you for cheering me on from the sidelines. To all those who have hiked or bimbled with me down the years, stirring words into ideas and tears into laughter, thank you. To my new friends at Gloucestershire Love Her Wild, especially Viv and The Rachel – soon I will be free to walk the talk too! Thank you.

Over the long years of recovery from post-viral fatigue, many people, too many to list, supported and helped me. Thank you for your professionalism and patience. I quite literally would not have recovered without you.

To my male friends who have suffered in their own way from the laminations of patriarchy – thank you for your friendship, for being feminists and for being 'Honorary Crones'. I hope it is a badge you wear with pride.

My thanks to Anna and Sara, who gave me sanctuary and a room with the most incredible view of the Small Isles to write my final chapters. To Doug and Gay, who made me feel at home when I needed one.

Finally, and most importantly, my heartfelt thanks and love to my family who have encouraged and supported me, even when their eyebrows were telling me that perhaps I was going a little cuckoo. To Liam and Danni, to my wise daughters Hannah and Kate and my glorious 'FIGOs', Florence, Iris, Grace and Olive. Thank you for all your love, care – and technology fixing! I love you all so much. Love who you are, honour and celebrate the unique you.

To my parents, sadly no longer here, whose post-war married life started out in a wood store, but your love and training in resilience sustains me now. Mum, just in case you are having a celestial read of this, and in keeping with tradition, I'll let you have the last word – 'There's no point getting old if you don't get artful!'

Thanks, Mum, thanks for everything.

May we all be artful.

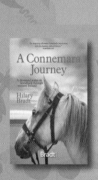
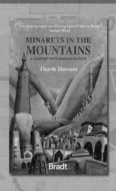
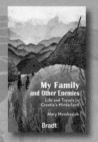
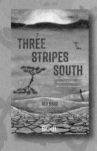
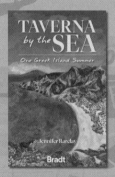
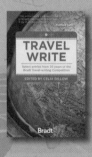

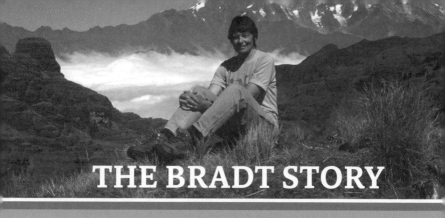

THE BRADT STORY

In the beginning

It all began in 1974 on an Amazon river barge. During an 18-month trip through South America, two adventurous young backpackers – Hilary Bradt and her then husband, George – decided to write about the hiking trails they had discovered through the Andes. *Backpacking Along Ancient Ways in Peru and Bolivia* included the very first descriptions of the Inca Trail. It was the start of a colourful journey to becoming one of the best-loved travel publishers in the world; you can read the full story on our website (bradtguides.com/ourstory).

Getting there first

Hilary quickly gained a reputation for being a true travel pioneer, and in the 1980s she started to focus on guides to places overlooked by other publishers. The Bradt Guides list became a roll call of guidebook 'firsts'. We published the first guide to Madagascar, followed by Mauritius, Czechoslovakia and Vietnam. The 1990s saw the beginning of our extensive coverage of Africa: Tanzania, Uganda, South Africa, and Eritrea. Later, post-conflict guides became a feature: Rwanda, Mozambique, Angola, and Sierra Leone, as well as the first standalone guides to the Baltic States following the fall of the Iron Curtain, and the first post-war guides to Bosnia, Kosovo and Albania.

Comprehensive – and with a conscience

Today, we are the world's largest independently owned travel publisher, with more than 200 titles. However, our ethos remains unchanged. Hilary is still keenly involved, and **we still get there first**: two-thirds of Bradt guides have no direct competition.

But we don't just get there first. Our guides are also known for being **more comprehensive** than any other series. We avoid templates and tick-lists. Each guide is a one-of-a-kind expression of an expert author's interests, knowledge and enthusiasm for telling it how it really is.

And a commitment to wildlife, conservation and respect for local communities has always been at the heart of our books. Bradt Guides was **championing sustainable travel** before any other guidebook publisher. We even have a series dedicated to Slow Travel in the UK, award-winning books that explore the country with a passion and depth you'll find nowhere else.

Thank you!

We can only do what we do because of the support of readers like you – people who value less-obvious experiences, less-visited places and a more thoughtful approach to travel. Those who, like us, take travel seriously.

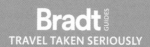

TRAVEL TAKEN SERIOUSLY